Making Psychotherapy More Effective with Unconscious Process Work

Making Psychotherapy More Effective with Unconscious Process Work is an essential text that seeks to educate readers on the astounding capabilities of unconscious intelligence to both gather information and engage in rapid cognition. By providing a comprehensive and easily understood overview of the recent research on unconscious processes, as well as clinical case material, this book provides readers with skills that will enable them to strategically engage these resources.

The first part of the book discusses the research-based principles that frame this growth-oriented approach towards psychotherapy. New discoveries about the surprising limitations of conscious self-governance force readers to reconsider the overall aim of psychotherapy. The second part explores several transtheoretical techniques, focusing on prediction, reimagining, mental contrasting, and incubated cognition. Case examples and key point summaries are used throughout, with the last chapter featuring reflective exercises. This book is essential reading for practicing psychotherapists, Ericksonian therapists, graduate students, and professors of psychotherapy.

Dan Short, PhD, is director of the Milton H. Erickson Institute of Phoenix and former Assistant Director for the Milton H. Erickson Foundation. He has authored several books and book chapters on Ericksonian Therapy and is leading the effort to document the core competencies of Ericksonian Therapy. Currently teaching Clinical Hypnosis at the Southwest College of Naturopathic Medicine, he conducts consultation groups for professionals in the Phoenix metropolitan area, provides supervision of professionals in the United States and abroad, and presents seminars and workshops as visiting faculty at institutes around the world. www.iamdrshort.com/book

Making Psychotherapy More Effective with Unconscious Process Work

Dan Short

Routledge
Taylor & Francis Group
NEW YORK AND LONDON

First published 2022
by Routledge
605 Third Avenue, New York, NY 10158

and by Routledge
2 Park Square, Milton Park, Abingdon, Oxon OX14 4RN

Routledge is an imprint of the Taylor & Francis Group, an informa business

Library of Congress Cataloging-in-Publication Data
A catalog record for this title has been requested

ISBN: 978-0-367-64967-8 (hbk)
ISBN: 978-0-367-64965-4 (pbk)
ISBN: 978-1-003-12720-8 (ebk)

DOI: 10.4324/9781003127208

Typeset in Bembo
by Taylor & Francis Books

Contents

Acknowledgments

In the Bantu language of Tanzania, Africa, there is a special saying, "Omwana taba womoi," which translates, "A child belongs not to one parent or home." As we say in Western societies—it takes a village. The greatest joy in writing this book has been my interactions with the people who participated in its creation: those clients who trusted me and shared the most vulnerable parts of themselves, thereby enriching my own humanity; the talented group of practitioners who spent many weeks helping me improve upon the original manuscript; and dedicated scholars and researchers, such as Donald Meichenbaum, Irving Kirsch, and John Kihlstrom, who took time to review aspects of my work. Most important to the creation of this book, or any other work of mine, is the caring and supportive homelife I enjoy with three extraordinary people: my wife Aimee, my son Trevor, and my daughter Elise. The three of them fill our home with infectious laughter, warm-hearted moments, and a beautiful enthusiasm for life.

The "villagers" most directly involved in the maturation of this work include Aimee Short, Elise LeLarge, Gem Mason, Helen Adrienne, Isabelle Prevot-Stimec, Maria Sole, Menaj Shamsaee, and Roxanna Erickson-Klein. During our weekly "book club" meetings, these individuals helped me improve upon the clarity, flow, and intellectual rigor of this book. I am also grateful to Richard Hill for contributing a foreword. I wish that everyone could be so fortunate in having the type of close and loyal friendships that continue to carry me forward. It is only with this type of support that any of us can truly flourish.

Foreword

Dan Short takes us on an exciting, albeit challenging, exploration of a topic that continues to be robustly discussed in clinical and academic circles—"the conscious" and "the unconscious." The book is the guide for a journey that winds us through the concepts, applications, and utilization of *unconscious process work*.

Short introduces us to the principal features of the landscape in the opening pages. The concepts of "unconscious problem-solving" and "self-organizing change" immediately resonated with me, as these are key elements in my own work and writing. Short has such a delightful writing style and thorough knowledge of the supporting literature that it feels natural and comfortable for a wide-ranging set of doorways to be established and opened: the important conscious subset of public and private; Freud's introduction of depth psychology; the fundamental principles of talk therapy; the frameworks of implicit perceptions and explicit expressions; and the problematic impacts of introspective therapy, including emotional flooding and shame. Each doorway is fundamentally important to both the practice of psychotherapy and the professional development of the psychotherapeutic practitioner.

Early in this book, my curiosity was piqued, and my sense of fascination was stimulated.

Conscious awareness is a curious thing. It is so common that it is often taken for granted as something simple and obvious. It is not. There are many names that need to be mentioned when discussing awareness without consciousness, and this book does not disappoint. William James, Frederick Myers, Pierre Janet, Boris Sidis, and Sigmund Freud are where we begin as Short takes us along a pathway that arrives at Milton Erickson.

In contrast to Freud, Erickson presented a new perspective that unconscious resources held the greatest potential for therapeutic change. Erickson's ideas expanded in the 1970s, especially during his collaboration with Ernest Rossi. After Erickson's death, Rossi continued developing our understanding of how to trust the unconscious as an effective and fertile ground for natural problem solving and for mind to body healing (Hill and Rossi 2018). Recent work by Joseph LeDoux and Richard Brown (2017) describes the natural process of creating a non-conscious representation of outer and inner stimuli before we make a second representation in our conscious awareness. This is encouraging support for the ideas that Short presents throughout this book. More importantly, it provides a parallel framework that contributes to our understanding of the case studies Short uses to illustrate the use of unconscious processing.

It is surprising that we place so much importance on our conscious states and our conscious awareness. So much of what emerges into conscious awareness begins in our nonconscious, automatic, and self-organizing processes. When teaching, I often use the simple example of that interesting thought that pops into our conscious awareness several times each day—I'm hungry. This idea becomes conscious after a host of complex activities have been active for an hour and a half or two. It involves production of hormones and peptides, changes in the activity of various parts of the viscera, activation of hunger-related areas of the sub-cortical brain, all resulting in the simple emergent feeling of being hungry. We don't even know what we are hungry for. Is it 3 mg of B6 or a teaspoon of folate? But when the need becomes conscious, we are prompted to activate our body to go to the fridge and get some food. It might be argued that consciousness is the latecomer to much of our experience and often only presents a somewhat club-fisted version of the deeper psycho-biological message. It is this second, conscious representation that turns on our executive network in the brain to produce a *task-positive response*. This is how we are able to survive. But there is, in my mind, little doubt that those aspects of mind that are not conscious do the lion's share of what is needed to keep us in good health and wellbeing. It is exactly the part of mind we need to engage to facilitate effective therapy.

To this end, Short takes us through a host of mental activities that I'm sure many of us are convinced are conscious processes and shows just how much we are mistaken, or, at least, we misunderstand. Although our cognitive processes are important and valuable to therapy and to daily life, it is the vast interplay of activity that occurs beneath the surface of consciousness that is doing the necessary preparatory work. Our unconscious is a place used by our self-preservation systems to hide many of those things that can do us harm. Our implicit world can be full of memories, emotional horrors, traumas, and deficits that are too much to deal with in the conscious space. Their effects are felt as emergent states that might include depression, anxiety, addictions, or social dysfunction. But, just like "I'm hungry," these conscious awarenesses, or what we often call symptoms, are blunt expressions of something far more complex, detailed, and nuanced. It is very hard to repair the damage to the kitchen by mowing the lawn, even though passersby might think that the house is well cared for and in good condition.

There are so many interesting things in this book that make reading it both enjoyable and educational. From Stroop tests to metaphors to the powerful effects of imagination, you will find that this journey will reveal something more than gold or gems. It will reveal more of you, your clients, and, I suggest, your life.

Richard Hill, MA, MEd, MBMSc, presents internationally on the topics of human dynamics, communications, the brain and the mind, and his specialty:

Curiosity & Possibility. He is past-President of the Global Association of Interpersonal Neurobiology Studies (GAINS), Education Director of The Science of Psychotherapy, Director of the Mindscience Institute, and Managing Editor of *The Science of Psychotherapy*.

Richard Hill

References

Hill, Richard, and Ernest L. Rossi. 2018. *The Practitioner's Guide to Mirroring Hands: A Client-Responsive Therapy That Facilitates Natural Problem-Solving and Mind-Body Healing.* Crown House Publishing Ltd.

LeDoux, Joseph E., and Richard Brown. 2017. "*A Higher-Order Theory of Emotional Consciousness.*" *Proceedings of the National Academy of Sciences* 114 (10): E2016–2025. https://doi.org/10.1073/pnas.1619316114.

1 What is Unconscious Process Work?

If the question for psychotherapy is how to best make use of a person's mental faculties, then the answer must include some activation of tacit knowledge, or what I call *unconscious process work*. Unconscious process work can seem mystical and improbable. Metaphorically, it is like lying down under the night sky and watching stationary stars pass by. You realize that during your moment of stillness the earth has moved you. In the following pages, we will see that conscious intention is a lesser thing that rides on much larger bodies of influence.

The best way I know to introduce an idea is to define it and then describe it in action. Within neuroscience, a distinction is often made between content versus process. Content relates to the storage of information, and process is the movement and transformation of information as it passes from one brain structure to another. Similarly, unconscious process work is the transformation of implicit content (e.g., memories, percepts, attitudes, emotions, expectations) in a way that affects the person's ongoing phenomenological experiences, thoughts, and actions.

To demonstrate, we begin with a case example from my clinical experience. It offers a minimalistic view of unconscious process work that does not involve complex techniques. By definition, techniques are the byproducts of principles. For depth of understanding, as you read the case example, search for underlying principles and ignore the technique. Because it was so individualized, I have rarely used this technique, but the same principles will be echoed on every page of this book (e.g., unconscious problem-solving and self-organizing change).

One of my first post-doctorate clients was a young woman who had read about Milton Erickson (1901–1980) and decided to seek out an Ericksonian therapist. Before ending her initial phone call, she asked, "Is it alright if I fax you a list of my concerns?"

The first thought that came to my mind was Erickson's admonishment to accept everything the client has to offer and then find some way to utilize it, which I did.

When her fax arrived, I was surprised to see that it was a full two pages filled with bullet-pointed items of intense concern. These included having a

DOI: 10.4324/9781003127208-1

pattern of dating abusive men, feeling intensely inferior to others around her, and being unable to recall much of her childhood.

When she came in for the first time, I greeted my client with her list in hand. It seemed the best way to utilize her list was to read it with her. After she sat and gave her consent, I conducted a slow, meticulous, word-for-word reading of her statements aloud. My recitation was so slow that it took half the session. During this time she did not speak, did not blink, and hardly seemed aware of anything else.

Shortly after I read the final item, she began to search for words to express her experience. Her hesitant response was, "It all seems so different when I listen to you read it. Hearing your voice describe my problems makes them seem different."

I asked her what she wanted to do with the rest of our time together. She said that she wanted to talk a little more about her boyfriend—how she met him and how he had treated her. This part of the session was more traditional, with her talking and me actively listening. Before she left, I asked her to say when she felt it would be the right time to return—the first thing to pop into her mind. She said that for some reason four weeks seemed right.

Four weeks later, she returned and was eager to tell me about her progress. She explained that in the past she had clung to abusive boyfriends until they eventually dumped her. She was always at the losing end. Now, for the first time, she had decided to end the relationship. She explained that after her therapy, she developed the strong feeling that he was not right for her. So, she moved out of his place and rented her own apartment.

This was a big move for her because she had never lived on her own—she had never experienced the feeling of being in charge of the space around her. As she explained, "I cannot say what made me decide to do this, but I realized that I need to discover who I am and that I cannot do that while I am with *this* guy."

She was absolutely thrilled with her new discoveries. As she said,

> I went to Target and bought red drapes! No one I know would approve of me hanging red drapes. But I like them! I think that red is my favorite color … It was such a wonderful sense of freedom. I bought a CD with Native American flute music. I was so happy sitting in my new apartment listening to my music with a candle burning. It is as if I am just now discovering what things I like.

In this case, most of the process work occurred outside of the client-therapist dialogue and beyond the margin of conscious review or understanding. To understand how this rapid change occurred for the client, we start with the classical definition of process work and then progress to a more modern, scientifically informed understanding of unconscious dynamics.

1.1 Traditional Process Work is Built on Freudian Principles

Hearing the words *process work* leads most to think of Sigmund Freud (1856–1939) and a therapeutic method that seeks to increase conscious awareness of unconscious processes (uncovering work). Indeed, the term first appeared in the 1970s when Jungian psychologist Arnold Mindell used it to describe his approach to increasing awareness of unconscious emotions and cognition. Mindell's transpersonal psychology sought to help people develop personal awareness and identify with repressed thoughts, emotions, and experiences that may negatively affect their everyday life.

In the context above, to "process an issue" means helping people integrate the psychological aftermath of a traumatic event within an autobiographical narrative. Most importantly, this narrative is coherent and can be expressed in words. As you read more about the evolution of this concept, keep in mind that we will soon turn in the opposite direction.

The paradigm underlying classical process work traces back to Sigmund Freud (1915), who divided all mental activity into two complementary forms of experience—primary processes and secondary processes. Simply put, primary process describes the discharge of biologically based instincts, such as the primitive urges for sex (eros) or aggression (thanatos). But biological drives alone are not enough to govern the actions of a complex organism. As Freud (1900) puts it,

> It will be rightly objected that an organization which was a slave to the pleasure principle and neglected the reality of the external world could not maintain itself alive for the shortest time, so that it could not have come into existence at all.
>
> (603)

Thus, Freud concluded there must be a secondary process, one that is capable of binding or regulating the flow of psychic energy as the organism seeks to reconcile itself with the consequences of engaging an external world.

Freud (1924, 306) used the terms *conscious* and *unconscious* nominally and spatially, with the unconscious being a mental location that acts as a repository, a "cauldron" of primitive wishes and impulses kept at bay and mediated within a medial level of awareness. This is the preconscious, the place where thought is initially formed as ideas pass from knowledge of thing-representations to word-representations (what non-Freudian theorists, such as Prince, referred to as the subconscious). Next, at the level of conscious awareness, word-based thought is used to allow for the displacement of small quantities of energy. In sum, psychological difficulties were viewed as pent-up energy that can be safely discharged during therapeutic dialogue.

These ideas formed the basis of the talking cure. Many decades since Freud, this same basic approach has been enshrined in the popular maxim "You have to name it to tame it." In other words, the effects of raw emotional energy become less intense when we can discuss our feelings with someone capable of empathetic understanding. Importantly, this view of process work places great emphasis on verbal expression (the client's words mediate change). Freud designed analytic therapy to be the antithesis of classical hypnotherapy (the hypnotist's words mediate change).

In contrast to classical process work, my client was never asked to describe her feelings, nor was her childhood mentioned. In contrast to traditional hypnotherapy, I did not offer any discernable suggestions for any specific change to occur. To recognize the principles at work, a paradigm shift is required.

1.2 Conscious Process Work Can Be Harmful

Freud is not the only one to argue for the importance of discussing our thoughts and feelings. From an academic perspective, cognitive scientists have found that conscious processing helps solidify new attitudes. Similarly, psychotherapy researcher Leslie Greenberg (2012) argues that a spoken (dialectical) synthesis of emotion and reason produces meaning. From this Jamesian perspective, emotion makes action possible while conscious organization adds coherence. Greenberg claims that without conscious articulation, the depth, range, and complexity of emotion cannot develop beyond its instinctual origins. For scholars such as Greenberg, emotional process work is always done at the conscious level of experience, symbolizing it with words and reflecting on it in order to create new narrative meaning. However, as with any set solution, its strength is its weakness.

Folk wisdom has long held that sometimes it is best not to "over think" certain experiences. The more complex and emotionally provocative the object of observation is, the more this seems to be true. Consequently, experiments in a wide variety of contexts have shown that attempts to put complex sensory experience into words impairs judgment and memory. Thus, there are times when words are not enough to capture the complexity of a phenomenological reality. The term used to describe this is *verbal overshadowing.*

This effect was first reported by Schooler and Englster-Schooler (1990). In this classic study, participants were asked to watch a video of a robbery and then either verbally describe the robber or engage in a distracting task. The result was that those who described the robber were less likely to correctly identify the individual in a lineup. In other words, putting an experience into words can result in failures of memory about that experience, whether it be the memory of a person's face, voice, or the color of an object. The effect occurs with a seemingly endless number of nonverbal perceptual stimuli. When conducting therapy, it is important to recognize that the client's own words can distort truth, even to the point of creating false memories.

An even more insidious problem is the distortion of spontaneity by conscious intention. This phenomenon has been named the *paradox of introspection.* While studying happiness, psychologists Schooler, Ariely, and Loewenstein (2003) found that the direct pursuit of positive internal states can produce a negative effect. What they found was that both the active monitoring of pleasure and the deliberate intention to enjoy an activity lead to decreased enjoyment. In other words, therapy clients who are encouraged to engage in *effortful introspection* with deliberate attempts to attain a greater sense of well-being may experience the paradoxical effect of becoming more and more discontent with their emotional disposition!

For both verbal overshadowing and effortful introspection, the negative effects disappear once a person reaches a certain level of expertise and proficiency. Thus, the reason therapists love to attend workshops that offer exciting new vocabulary and introspective exercises might be because most are highly proficient in these skills. Clients, on the other hand, may not be prepared to reap the same rewards.

A third problem is emotional flooding—harm caused by excess emotion. This unpleasant experience can produce lasting negative effects. I witnessed this early in my career at a training event. A colleague came out of a psychodynamic therapy group disoriented and in a state of intense emotional distress. She could barely speak and did not know where to go. While the psychodynamic technique certainly achieves its goal of intensifying the patient's emotional arousal and uncovering old wounds, it can also lead to horrible feelings of shame and failure. This happens when all responsibility for maintaining a productive exchange is thrust upon a struggling client.

As for my friend, I walked her back to her room and suggested she could find privacy and safety there, especially in the bathtub with warm water all the way up to her neck and all the lights off. I called it a "return to the womb experience" (her mother had committed suicide when she was 14 years of age). The next day she smiled and told me she had an amazing return to the womb experience.

Clients become emotionally flooded when pushed too far too fast. As I learned while working in the field of domestic violence, the consequences of emotional flooding can be significant. Those who become overly angry may leave therapy and harm themselves or others. Similarly, therapists who work with complex trauma are aware that clients who uncover too much repressed emotional pain may sink into a long-term state of clinical depression. And as with any disorder, those who experience excessive shame may never return to therapy.

Wurmser (1981) observed that shame tends to follow the exposure of something we would have preferred to keep private. This shame can then lead to other intense emotions, such as demoralization or rage. As an interesting example, I had a client comment on the superficial nature of his relationship with his mother, whom he did not trust. As a 35-year-old man, he was still angry at his mother for something that happened when he was in middle school. When I asked him to explain, he said that he had really liked a girl in his class and told his mother. His mother mentioned it to a close friend, who then went and told the mother of the girl. A little later, when the teens were at a bowling alley, the girl approached my client to find out if it was true that he liked her. He felt such sudden and intense shame that he walked off and never again spoke to her. Consequently, he decided to never again trust his mother. In this instance, and many like it, the shame reaction was covered by subsequent emotions (anger and disgust).

This same type of avoidance can be triggered within therapy. After talking to colleagues, I know that I am not the only therapist to have a client open up and reveal compelling personal secrets, only to never return. The promise of confidentiality is not enough to ensure that shame will not prevail.

This prompts the question, When should something be declared out loud or left private? According to Donald Nathanson (1994, 319) "uncovering therapies produce an 'arena of shame.'" I have heard some equate it to psychological nudity. When conducting depth work, if the suddenly exposed emotions have been kept private from the individual's own conscious awareness, then the result can be sudden and intense shame.

Unless there is room for maintaining one's privacy, exploratory work could result in avoiding important content or quitting therapy. As Nathanson (2000) puts it, clients who are already overwhelmed with negative self-images cannot stand any new emotional insight because it only brings more shame. Accordingly, Erickson would instruct his clients to only tell him the things they are ready for him to know and to keep the rest private. Of course, this creates a moving target. The more his clients would share, the more comfortable they became with sharing just a little bit more. Erickson's general strategy was to create an atmosphere of protection and respectful attentiveness.

When a client suddenly becomes silent, this can be indicative of shame. Though the shame may not be consciously experienced, the body and behavior speak to the deeper affective experience. Like jealousy, shame is often concealed by anger. Under such circumstances, a traditional analytic posture (wait in silent neutrality) is not helpful. I had one client complain that a therapist spent the entire therapy hour sitting in silence with a blank expression. In addition to quitting therapy, he said he wanted to punch her in the face.

Whenever a client becomes emotionally disoriented or starts to experience the effects of shame, my tendency is to take responsibility for initiating a meaningful exchange. I take pressure off the client by moving the focus of attention back to myself and the question of whether I am performing adequately.

For example, I might say to a client, "I am not certain what to say. I need a little more time to process what we have been discussing. Please excuse me if I am silent for a while. My unconscious mind is working on something." As the client sits and watches me gazing toward the ground in a state of quiet reflection, it primes (prompts) the client with same behavior. Soon, the indirect suggestion for process work takes effect, and the client declares, "I just realized something important …." Although this technique also involves the use of silence, as does the analytic posture, it operates under the principle of protection and thereby shields the client from shame.

Social scientists have concluded that people are foremost relational beings, which means that we (unconsciously) define ourselves, and our circumstances, in large part by others' responses to us. This is why it is helpful for those who are struggling to find a wise authority figure with whom they can become emotionally invested. With kind, empathetic engagement there is a greater sense of safety and personal significance. If the client's unconscious sentiment could be heard, it might sound something like, "This doctor wants to be with me and thinks that my experiences are important!" This positive relational experience helps reduce insecurity and negative affect.

When we look at process work within the context of traditional therapies, we clearly see the importance of being known by others. The acknowledgement and validation that comes from a capable therapist can have powerful emotional effects. But this does not mean that every client needs to consciously process and disclose deep content. As demonstrated in the opening case example, a carefully crafted therapy session can include conscious as well as unconscious process work.

1.3 Positive Depth Psychology Emphasizes Unconscious Capabilities

For most of recorded human history, only the concepts of conscious thought and intentional behavior existed. Then in the 1800s, three very different developments—hypnotism, parapsychology, and evolutionary theory—all pointed to the possibility of mental processes that were operating outside the margins of conscious awareness. As scientists and clinicians began to investigate the former, new theories were developed to explain the experience of non-volitional behavior (suggestion effects), alleged psychic abilities (subliminal perception), and automaticity (genetic transmission of behavior).

Although the public at large only knows Freudian depth psychology, earlier in the nineteenth century there was another more positive theory of unconscious operations. The philosopher Eduard von Hartmann (1869) and the philologist Frederick W. Myers (1886) both wrote about the superior abilities of unconscious intelligence (Gurney et al., 1886). While Freud acknowledges having been influenced by Hartmann, James gave special attention to articles published by Myers (1892), who argued that the phenomena of Spiritualism (e.g., automatic writing) were not caused by an external intelligence but instead by an internal intelligence operating outside of awareness. Speaking of Myers, James (1902, 229) described his theories as "the most important step forward that has occurred in psychology since I have been a student of that science." As James (1902) describes it:

> there is not only the consciousness of the ordinary field, with its usual center and margin, but in addition thereto in the shape of a set of memories, thoughts, and feelings which are extra-marginal and outside of the primary consciousness altogether, but yet must be classed as conscious facts of some sort, able to reveal their presence by unmistakable signs.
>
> (229)

With this endorsement, Myers's theory became influential and was cited by several pioneers in clinical psychology, such as Pierre Janet (who developed the clinical concept of engaging the subconscious mind), Theodore Flournoy (whose concept of a prospective element in the unconscious had a significant impact on Carl Jung) and Boris Sidis (one of the early architects of clinical psychology in America and author of the seminal textbook, *The Psychology of Suggestion: A Research into the Subconscious Nature of Man and Society* [1889]).

A key point is that Myers's concept of subliminal intelligence was more expansive than Freud's subsequent formulation of an animalistic unconscious. According to Myers (1892, 350), "a stream of consciousness flows on within us, at a level beneath the threshold of ordinary waking life … this consciousness embraces unknown powers of which these hypnotic phenomena give us the first sample, the scattered indications."

Similarly, James (1902) argued that the presence of unconscious intelligence also helped explain many religious phenomena, such as hearing instructions from God, being controlled by outside spirits, or experiencing faith healing. As outlined by Janet (1925), Myers's subliminal intelligence was not only capable of subliminal perception and regulation of autonomic processes, but also of engaging in higher cognition, such as goal formation, moral decision making, tracking time, and making complex predictions. Janet also credits Myers with the argument that these unconscious tendencies exist in all of us at all times. In sum, Myers argued that we are more intellectually capable than we can consciously know.

Like the modern positive psychology movement, positive depth psychology examines the vital contribution of unconscious processes to everyday life. From this perspective, this mysterious part of the mind is seen as having processing capabilities that are equal, if not superior, to conscious reason. In the words of William James (1982, 91), unconscious processes are "the organizing center of personality." While James (1890) believed that the terms *thought* and *emotion* should be restricted to descriptions of conscious awareness, he also argued for the intellectual capabilities of unconscious problem-solving, describing them as "far wiser than and superior to that of normal, waking, rational awareness" (Taylor, 1982, 91).

These ideas seem to have formed the foundation for the clinical innovations of another iconic figure, Milton Erickson. Rather than embracing Freud's wildly popular description of the unconscious as something that is irrational and destructive, Erickson embraced a more positive view of unconscious capabilities.

In fact, Erickson took the Jamesian model a step further by arguing that unconscious processes include superior cognitive skills (as used in goal setting and problem-solving) and superior abilities for mentally representing and working toward the integration of emotional experiences. As Erickson (1948, 577) stated early in his career, "Good unconscious understandings allowed to become conscious before a conscious readiness exists will result in conscious resistance, rejection, repression and even the loss, through repression, of unconscious gains." This brings us back to Freud's (1915) observation that some events and desires were too frightening or painful for his patients to acknowledge. Thus, Erickson accepted Freud's theory of repression, which has since been demonstrated in well-controlled studies (for an example, see Williams, 1994).

What makes Erickson's perspective fundamentally different from traditional psychotherapy is his acceptance of the limitations of conscious awareness and his utilization of unconscious processes for the therapeutic endeavor.

Erickson believed that conscious working memory is inherently less resilient to toxic emotional states than the working memory that operates at purely unconscious levels. For example, while describing his use of unconscious process work for trauma therapy, Erickson explains, "It may be too painful a thing for her ever to recognize consciously." (Erickson and Haley, 1985, 4) Thus, extremely toxic ideas should be processed unconsciously so that their impact can be mitigated prior to emerging into conscious awareness.

Erickson believed that this approach to process work is not only good therapy but also an ethical obligation. As Erickson explains, "You protect that patient. You're protecting the conscious mind by keeping that self-understanding unconscious." (Erickson et al., 1976, 256) Thus, rather than searching for past events and seeking to bring these painful or overwhelming experiences into conscious awareness (insight therapy), Erickson's method utilizes automatic coping strategies that are already in play. As soon as a cooperative, collaborative interpersonal exchange is established, these automatic strategies are elaborated and applied toward some productive end.

For example, coping strategies might include repression, denial, social isolation, somatization, or a purely symbolic representation of the problem situation. As illustrated in the case description at the start of this chapter, this person's distillation of the problem situation was in written form, which allowed me to recognize its importance and bring it into therapy. But why did she need to present her problems to me in written form prior to our face-to-face meeting?

Thinking of your own life experiences (perhaps a love note written to a crush or a painful apology), it is easy to recognize that sometimes we can manage to put into writing something that we cannot say out loud directly to another person. That is because speaking our most private thoughts while looking someone else in the eyes greatly intensifies the emotional reality of the experience. If a client is asked to share private information in narrative form (tell me your story), the emotional arousal is intensified still further—perhaps to the point of emotional flooding.

My tactic was to utilize the client's coping strategy (her list) and only speak her words as she had written them, but in a slow, careful, and non-emotional manner. It was this extra time (30 minutes of slow recitation) that provided space for her unconscious to begin processing the deeper meaning of the ideas. Thus, *unconscious process work moves in the opposite direction of conscious process work*. The therapy began with a conscious definition of the problem(s), but in the absence of conversation, all was ceded to unconscious processing.

My client was primed to respond with process work by the nature of the setting (a therapist's office). Because I did not engage her in a back-and-forth dialogue, no demands were placed on her conscious resources. Thus, mental energy was freed up for use by unconscious processes.

Due to the timing of the apparent changes that occurred for this client, it is reasonable to assume that the therapeutic process work was beneficial. Yet it is equally possible that her progress was caused by some other, unknown variable. As we search for ideas we can trust, the conceptual foundation for this book will be checked against a large body of well-established, empirical research.

1.4 Understanding the Science/Practice Divide

Initially, Freudian depth psychology, which was foundational to twentieth-century psychotherapeutics, was summarily rejected by those conducting research. Ignoring James's enthusiastic embrace of unconscious functionality, researchers followed the lead of William Wundt (1832–1920), who rejected making unconscious mental processes a topic of scientific psychology. These foundational differences created a mistrust between researchers and clinicians that remains palpable to this day.

The story of this schism begins in 1904 when William James triggered a fierce debate within the academic community. The intellectual dilemmas he exposed left psychologists scrambling to determine what exactly is the science of mind and whether such a thing can even exist. According to Robert Wozniak, James's (1904) exigent philosophical article "Does Consciousness Exist?" questioned:

> Was consciousness a metaphysical entity or simply a particular sort of relationship toward objects into which portions of pure experience enter? Was consciousness a stream of experience, a kind of awareness, or thought? Was it an adaptive function or a composite of states; an energetic by-product of neurophysiological process, another name for associative learning, a form of arrested movement, a regulator of future adaptation, or simply another way of describing "self"?
>
> (Wozniak, 1997)

The answer to this collective existential crisis came in the person of John B. Watson (1878–1958), the father of behaviorism. Watson (1913) blamed psychology's failure to "make its place in the world as an undisputed natural science" on the "esoteric" nature of its introspective method (asking people to report on their psychological experiences) (163). Rejecting all data based on self-report as well as the use of consciousness as an interpretive standard, Watson urged psychologists to adopt behavior as their unit of analysis.

Watson convincingly argued that the task of psychology should be to manipulate the external stimulus environment and objectively measure the subject's responses. Standardization and replicability were prized above any consideration of phenomenology, even that which is central to human existence, such as feelings of love or imagination and creativity.

1.5 Science "Discovers" the Unconscious

It was not until the fall of behaviorism and the 1960s cognitive revolution that mental processes, such as apprehension, primary memory, attention, and imagery, once again became a legitimate topic of study in scientific psychology. Almost immediately, researchers found it necessary to make a distinction of one kind or another between conscious and unconscious processing. Now the term *unconscious* has been redefined in modern studies as all the mental processes that are not experienced by a person but that give rise to his or her thoughts, choices, emotions, and behavior (Schacter et al., 2011, 188).

I say redefined because its contemporary use is as an adjective that describes a wide array of functional capabilities, rather than a nominal term that points to a region of the mind. Even Freud (1915) seemed uneasy with his categorization of "the unconscious":

> let us state the important, though inconvenient, fact that the attribute of being unconscious is only one feature that is found in the psychical and is by no means sufficient fully to characterize it. There are psychical acts of very varying value which yet agree in possessing the characteristic of being unconscious.
>
> (172)

Drew Westen (1999) explains the modern conceptualization well, writing,

> we do not group a class of cognitive processes together and call them "the cognitive," any more than we speak of "the efficient," "the adaptive," or "the distressing." Nor should we lump a large set of processes together and call them "the unconscious," as if they all do the same thing, serve the same function, or operate on the same principles. We should instead speak of unconscious processes.
>
> (1095)

One of the most familiar examples of an unconscious process is the formation of conditioned responses following a stimulus-response pairing (associative learning), resulting in behaviors that operate automatically and outside of awareness. A second widely accepted example is the presence of instinctual behaviors, which are activated by situational factors and often operate outside intentional control.

Following the lead of depth psychology, new studies have revealed a more complex and dynamic set of interactions between numerous systems.

As Elizabeth Phelps (2004) has pointed out, the unconscious emerging from research is routinely involved in affect, motivation, and even executive control and metacognition. Unconscious processes can sometimes include elements of conscious awareness, effortful processing (requiring working memory), intentionality and self-evaluation, as well as goal setting, self-regulation, and adaptive learning (Bargh, 1994; Melnikoff and Bargh, 2018).

What eventually came to be recognized was that all major mental processes and states can be *unconscious* (occurring outside of conscious awareness) and/or *implicit* (occurring automatically without attention or intention). Thus, the modern unconscious emerged as an unavoidable dimension in nearly every field of inquiry in psychology, cognitive neuroscience, behavioral economics, and the humanities. For example, in the field of cognitive linguistics, the study of generative grammar seeks to better understand the linguistic structures below the level of conscious awareness, such as presupposition and metaphoric meaning. In research on motor control and on language production, the conscious aspects of voluntary action and action monitoring are contrasted with unconscious aspects of motor programming, which includes the implicit learning of motor sequences. In modern perception research, psychophysical measurement continues to make the distinction of supraliminal versus subliminal stimulation.

In the study of attention, the term "attentional awareness" is often contrasted with unconscious, "pre-attentive" processing. Research on the social science of persuasion makes a distinction between central processing versus peripheral route (with central processing being more conscious and deliberate, while the peripheral route relies on implicit processing). And in memory research, the distinction is made between declarative memory (explicit processing) and procedural memory (implicit processing). Lastly, in various reincarnations of Freud's dual-process typology, several fields now contrast "automatic" processing (type 1), which tends to be associated with unconscious mechanisms, versus "controlled" processing (type 2), which tends to be associated with consciousness. Of all these, the research that has gathered the most attention is the work with subliminal perception, priming, and decision-making—specifically the study of heuristics and biases.

With this rapidly expanding body of research, it has become nearly impossible to ignore the significant role of unconscious processes in day-to-day human behavior. Regardless of the terminology used to describe it, the difference between conscious and unconscious processes is an inescapable contrast.

One of the most important discoveries of modern research into unconscious cognition is that all thought and behavior get their start at the level of unconscious processing. This revelation seems to have been anticipated by the German philosopher Arthur Schopenhauer (1788–1860), who was the first person to theorize about unconscious cognition. Schopenhauer (1851) wrote:

> One might almost believe that half of our thinking takes place unconsciously. … I have familiarized myself with the factual data of a

> theoretical and practical problem; I do not think about it again, yet often a few days later the answer to the problem will come into my mind entirely from its own accord; the operation which has produced it, however, remains as much a mystery to me as that of an adding-machine: what has occurred is, again, unconscious rumination.
>
> (123–124)

Perhaps because the entire scientific enterprise is based on efforts to capitalize on conscious deliberation and critical thought; the idea of an unconscious intelligence has been reflexively rejected by academia. However, during the last thirty years a paradigm shift has occurred. Not only have social psychologists, such as John Kihlstrom (1987; Khilstrom et al., 2000), argued for a cognitive unconscious and an emotional unconscious; now there is controlled experimentation showing unconscious preferences and values, questions, and conclusions that together form the foundation for unconscious motives and goals (high-level cognition).

Confirmation of this principle forced academia to abandon a central premise of cognitive psychology in the 1970s, which was that higher mental processes were almost entirely under conscious, executive control. Given technological improvements from 1980 onwards (such as brain imaging techniques), researchers discovered unconscious processes not only support but also inform our most sophisticated mental activities. As Ran Hassin (2013) argues, unconscious processes can perform the same fundamental, high-level functions that conscious processes can perform.

With these conceptual advances, John Bargh (2019) has argued that psychological science has reached a unique point in history. Only recently have all three of the past century's most important competing schools of thought converged on a single, empirically supported construct. Bargh believes that the elegance of modern research on unconscious processes is its ability to combine the most important aspects of Freudian psychology, behaviorism, and cognitive psychology.

According to Bargh, current research clearly supports Freud's position that many important affective, motivational, and behavioral phenomena operate without the person's awareness or conscious intention. This same body of research also supports the position of behaviorism that unconscious processes are often triggered by events, people, situational settings, and other external stimuli. And, in keeping with cognitive psychology, it has been found that these external stimuli exert their effect through the automatic activation of internal mental representations and processes. These new developments in social cognitive research have been described by Hassin and others as the New Unconscious (Hassin et al., 2004).

1.6 Process Work is Problem-solving

In the past, there has been some debate over whether psychotherapy most appropriately focuses on emotional coping and affect regulation, or whether it should focus on problem-solving and direct efforts to change those factors that have created emotional distress (Lazarus and Folkman 1984). Thus, when considering the case example at the opening of the chapter, it is interesting to ask which of these was prioritized. The answer seems to be both.

Rather than thinking of emotional or autobiographical process work as being mutually exclusive to practical problem-solving, it is helpful to think of it as a pre-deliberative stage in the problem-solving process. As William James (1890) puts it, emotion prepares us for action. Later, we will examine how the process of problem-solving can be broken down into a deliberative stage (planning) and an implemental stage (executing action), each with its own distinct mindset. When I say that emotional process work is pre-deliberative, what I mean is that emotion shapes how we think about our problems, and it motivates us to action. As seen in the opening case example, once the stage is set, decisive action is likely to follow.

The findings of modern cognitive science support the possibility that unconscious process work was what enabled my client to emerge into an entirely new system of intellectual, emotional, and behavioral realities. This includes research that specifically addresses unconscious aspects of working memory as well as unconscious self-monitoring and self-regulation. This evidence suggests that during therapy my client was involved in a re-examination of the meaning of old memories and emotions, without conscious awareness.

An interesting challenge that all experts face while reading about the powerful influence of unconscious mental activity is how we reconcile our dependency on academic knowledge (as a source of authority) with the obvious limitations of conscious resources. A grave error in Freudian analysis was the assumption that the therapist, as an informed authority, could make perfectly objective interpretations while the patient presumably languished under the effects of his or her unconscious conflicts.

Therefore, as you read through this material and think about what it may mean for the people you work with, also keep in mind your own humble position as someone who is equally influenced by powerful unconscious forces. While conducting process work with the client, the ideal scenario is one in which your own unconscious processes are problem-solving the task of meeting the client's needs, both conscious and unconscious.

The thoughts of Michael Polanyi (1891–1976), a Hungarian-British polymath who made important theoretical contributions to chemistry, economics, and philosophy, provide a perfect encapsulation not only of this chapter but for the book as a whole: we know much more than we can tell.

Polanyi (1958) made this statement while introducing the concept of tacit knowledge, which is the skills, ideas, and experiences that people have, but they are not codified in cognition and thus are difficult to express. As a result, people are often not fully aware of the knowledge they possess or how it can be valuable to themselves and others. The best way to share tacit knowledge is through personal encounters that are characterized by collaborative interactions and trust (Goffin and Koners 2011)—the stuff of psychotherapy. Thus, if a person relies entirely on conscious knowledge for individual problem-solving, then the tacit knowledge gleaned from a lifetime of learning is lost. The point to take from this chapter is that unconscious process work is a strategic problem-solving methodology that places unconscious abilities in the lead position during tandem work with conscious intelligence. Furthermore, the point to take from this entire book is the pivotal role of unconscious processes during any psychological endeavor. As stated by William James over a century ago, "the subconscious is not only the most important problem of psychology, it is the problem" (quoted in Prince, 1912, 162).

Chapter 1 Key Points

- Unconscious process work does not require conscious insight. It also does not require trance states or suggestions for change. Instead, it is an exercise of unconscious creativity and personal problem-solving (self-organizing change).
- Conscious process work can be harmful, leading to emotional flooding, shame, or interference with spontaneous, intuitive behavior.
- Unconscious intelligence has processing capabilities that are in some ways superior to conscious reason (e.g., intuitive problem-solving). But there are also unique advantages to conscious intelligence (e.g., science).
- The contemporary science of unconscious processes combines the most important aspects of Freudian psychology, behaviorism, and cognitive psychology. The methodology of unconscious process work draws on all three of these as well as Ericksonian hypnotherapy.
- People are often unaware of the knowledge they possess and how to utilize it while problem-solving their greatest challenges.

References

Bargh, John A. 1994. "The Four Horsemen of Automaticity: Awareness, Efficiency, Intentions and Control." In *Handbook of Social Cognition*, edited by R. Wyer and T. Srull, 1–40. Hillsdale, NJ: Lawrence Erlbaum Associates.

Bargh, John A. 2019. "The Modern Unconscious." *World Psychiatry* 18 (2): 225–226. doi:10.1002/wps.20625.

Erickson, Milton H. 1948. "Hypnotic Psychotherapy." *Medical Clinics of North America* 32 (3): 571–583. doi:10.1016/S0025-7125(16)35675-9.

Erickson, Milton H., and Jay Haley. 1985. *Conversations with Milton H. Erickson, M. D., Vol. I: Changing Individuals*. 1st edition. San Diego: Triangle Press.

Erickson, Milton H., Ernest L. Rossi, and Sheila I. Rossi. 1976. "Hypnotic Realities: The Induction of Clinical Hypnosis and Forms of Indirect Suggestion." In *Hypnotic Realities: The Induction of Clinical Hypnosis and Forms of Indirect Suggestion*. Vol. 10. Phoenix, AZ: Milton H. Erickson Foundation Press.

Freud, Sigmund. (1900) 1966. "The Interpretation Of Dreams." In *The Basic Writings of Sigmund Freud*, translated and edited by A. A. Brill, 181–468. New York: Random House.

Freud, Sigmund. 1915. "The Unconscious." *SE* 14: 159–215.
Freud, Sigmund. 1924. *A General Introduction to Psychoanalysis*. Translated by Joan Riviere. Library of Alexandria.
Goffin, Keith, and Ursula Koners. 2011. "Tacit Knowledge, Lessons Learnt, and New Product Development." *Journal of Product Innovation Management* 28 (2): 300–318. doi:10.1111/j.1540-5885.2010.00798.x.
Greenberg, Leslie. 2012. "Emotions, the Great Captains of Our Lives: Their Role in the Process of Change in Psychotherapy." *American Psychologist* 67 (8): 697–707. doi:10.1037/a0029858.
Gurney, Edmund, Frederic W. H. Myers, and Frank Podmore. 1886. *Phantasms of the Living*. Cambridge: Cambridge University Press.
Hartmann, Eduard von. (1869) 1946. *Philosophy of the Unconscious: Speculative Results According to the Inductive Method of Physical Science*. New Edition, in One Volume. London: Kegan Paul, Trench, Trubner & Co. Ltd.
Hassin, Ran R. 2013. "Yes It Can: On the Functional Abilities of the Human Unconscious." *Perspectives on Psychological Science* 8 (2): 195–207. doi:10.1177/1745691612460684.
Hassin, Ran R., James S. Uleman, and John A. Bargh, eds. 2004. *The New Unconscious*. Oxford: Oxford University Press.
James, William. (1890) 1927. *The Principles of Psychology*, Vol. I–II. New York: Henry Holt.
James, William. (1902) 1917. *The Varieties of Religious Experience*. New York: Longmans, Green & Co.
James, William. 1904. "Does 'Consciousness' Exist?" *The Journal of Philosophy, Psychology, and Scientific Methods* 1 (18): 477–491. doi:10.2307/2011942.
Janet, Pierre. 1925. *Psychological Healing: A Historical and Clinical Study*. New York: Macmillan.
Kihlstrom, J. F. 1987. "The Cognitive Unconscious." *Science* 237 (4821): 1445–1452. doi:10.1126/science.3629249.
Kihlstrom, John F., Shelagh Mulvaney, Betsy A.Tobias, and Irene P. Tobis. 2000. "The Emotional Unconscious." In *Cognition and Emotion*, edited by Eric Eich, John F. Kihlstrom, Gordon H. Bower, Joseph P. Forgas, and Paula M. Niedenthal, 30–86. Oxford: Oxford University Press.
Lazarus, Richard, and Susan Folkman. 1984. *Stress, Appraisal, and Coping*. New York: Springer Publishing Company.
Melnikoff, David E., and John A. Bargh. 2018. "The Mythical Number Two." *Trends in Cognitive Sciences* 22 (4): 280–293. doi:10.1016/j.tics.2018.02.001.
Myers, Frederick W. (1892) 1976. *Subliminal Consciousness*. New York: Ayer Co Pub.
Nathanson, Donald L. 1994. *Shame and Pride: Affect, Sex, and the Birth of the Self*. New York: W. W. Norton & Company.
Nathanson, Donald L. 2000. "A Conversation with Donald Nathanson | Behavior Online." *Behavior Online* (blog). March 18. https://behavior.net/2000/03/a-conversation-with-donald-nathanson.
Phelps, Elizabeth A. 2004. "The Interaction of Emotion and Cognition: The Relation Between the Human Amygdala and Cognitive Awareness." In *The New Unconscious*, edited by Ran R. Hassin, James S. Uleman, and John A. Bargh, 61–76. Oxford: Oxford University Press.
Polanyi, Michael. (1958) 2012. *Personal Knowledge: Towards a Post-Critical Philosophy*. London: Routledge.

Prince, Morton. 1912. *The Unconscious: The Fundamentals of Human Personality, Normal and Abnormal.* New York: Macmillan.

Schacter, Daniel, Daniel Gilbert, Daniel Wegner, and Bruce M. Hood. 2011. *Psychology: European Edition.* New York: Macmillan International Higher Education.

Schooler, Jonathan W., Dan Ariely, and George Loewenstein. 2003. "The Pursuit and Monitoring of Happiness Can Be Self-Defeating." In *The Psychology of Economic Decisions*, edited by Isabelle Brocas and Juan D. Carrillo, 41–70. Oxford: Oxford University Press.

Schooler, Jonathan W., and Tonya Y. Engstler-Schooler. 1990. "Verbal Overshadowing of Visual Memories: Some Things Are Better Left Unsaid." *Cognitive Psychology* 22 (1): 36–71. doi:10.1016/0010-0285(90)90003-M.

Schopenhauer, Arthur. (1851) 2014. *Essays and Aphorisms.* London: Penguin.

Taylor, Eugene. 1982. *William James on Exceptional Mental States: The 1896 Lowell Lectures.* New York: Scribner.

Watson, John B. 1913. "Psychology as the Behaviorist Views It." *Psychological Review* 20 (2): 158–177. doi:10.1037/h0074428.

Westen, Drew. 1999. "The Scientific Status of Unconscious Processes: Is Freud Really Dead?" *Journal of the American Psychoanalytic Association* 47 (4): 1061–1106. doi:10.1177/00030651990470404.

Williams, Linda Meyer. 1994. "What Does It Mean to Forget Child Sexual Abuse?: A Reply to Loftus, Garry, and Feldman (1994)." *Journal of Consulting and Clinical Psychology* 62 (6): 1182–1186. doi:10.1037/0022-006X.62.6.1182.

Wozniak, Robert H. 1997. "Theoretical Roots of Early Behaviorism: Functionalism, the Critique of Introspection, and the Nature of Evolution and Consciousness." http://bascom.brynmawr.edu/psychology/rwozniak/theory.html.

Wurmser, Léon. 1981. *The Mask of Shame.* Baltimore, MD: Johns Hopkins University Press.

2 Perception and Memory

In this chapter, we will examine the domain of perception in its broadest sense. This includes conscious as well as unconscious perceptions and supraliminal as well as subliminal stimuli. Because this book is written for clinicians, I begin with Freudian concepts from which current western psychological approaches have evolved. As Blakey Vermeule (2015) poetically states,

> nowadays, psychoanalysis stands in much the same relation to academic mind science as paganism once stood to early Christianity. The new gods have built gleaming cathedrals on the ruins of the old gods' temples and the old gods have been made into the new devils.
>
> (467)

In other words, while the science of mind has changed a great deal since Freud, his ideas still serve as a point of reference. With the benefit of modern research capabilities, we will see how much more complex human perception is than was previously imagined.

I will begin with an example of behavior that most people have encountered, but perhaps without understanding the reasons behind it. This occurred during graduate training when I was studying counseling. It was late at night, and I had just left a two-hour group psychotherapy session led by one of the doctoral students. During group, I noticed a student glaring at me. She looked angry, though I had done nothing to her. This type of thing happens. One person in a crowd will decide not to like you for no apparent reason.

After leaving for the parking lot, this woman caught up with me at a spot to the side of the building where there were no lights or other students. With a serious look on her face, she said, "I want you to know that I spent most of the session trying to decide why I hate you—why I have so much anger that I want to kill you."

She paused and then continued, "It is only now that I realize what it is. It's your shirt! It's that white collar around your neck (the rest of the t-shirt was solid black). It looks like something a priest would wear." Curious, I inquired, "You went to Catholic school?" She had, so I changed the subject, and we had a pleasant talk as I walked her to her car.

DOI: 10.4324/9781003127208-2

This event occurred before news of the Catholic priest sex scandals emerged, but with her fixation on my collar, I was able to connect the dots. Outside, her anger had switched to trust. But this was not the case in the therapy room, when the reasons for her emotional reaction were only known to implicit perception. At that moment, her reaction seemed random—even to her.

Events that appear to be random may simply reflect our inability to consciously perceive the details of the processes involved. In the case above, the processes seem to include: unconscious perception, repressed memory, transference, and an instinctual urge to eliminate one's enemies. As evolutionary functionalism argues, human behavior is never random.

As an analogy, think about tossing a pair of dice and rolling a 12. Is that outcome random? If you were hoping for a 7, you will consider it random or bad luck. But, in fact, the roller of the dice orchestrates the outcome by means of pitch, velocity, timing of release, placement of each die in the hand, etc. It seems random because conscious introspection is not equipped to track and manage these details. As professionals, we are obliged to reconcile our actions in terms of reliable skill sets rather than random chance. Unfortunately, an introspective study of our craft cannot highlight the nuances of unconscious behavior. This requires the powerful lens of science.

The spectacular achievement by modern researchers of unconscious processes is the new capacity to observe and measure interactions between perception, memory, and emotion without having to depend on the subject's conscious awareness and introspection. Scientists can now consider details of unconscious processing not normally codified in cognitive awareness.

One of the most widely accepted findings from the research is that most of human behavior reflects unconscious processes, some of which are executed automatically and some of which are produced by implicit learning and thought (Kihlstrom, 2013). This invisible hand applies to virtually every area of psychological functioning: starting with perception and including memory, cognition, emotion, attitudes, and motivation (Westen, 1999; Wilson, 2004). In other words, it is unconscious mental activity that makes daily functioning possible. The reason for this large role is immediately evident when we compare the capacity of conscious versus unconscious perception.

As for the biological science of perception, most conservative estimates suggest that our senses deliver around 11 million pieces of information to our brains every second. The impulses carrying this information can travel as fast as 100,000 mph. From all of that, conscious awareness gleans approximately forty bits (.000004%), which is processed much more slowly (100 mph at best). This is the same as comparing the size of the African continent to Disneyland or the speed of a rocket to a turtle. In other words, consciousness can only deal with a very small percentage of all incoming information. All the rest is processed without awareness.

Freud was correct to assume that conscious awareness was only the tip of the iceberg, though unconscious mental activity is much more massive than his analogy suggests. However, Freud incorrectly equated unconscious processes with primitive instincts. Additionally, he assumed that the only reason primitive urges remain unconscious is to protect individuals from experiencing anxiety and distress. In contrast, the modern view of the adaptive unconscious, as described by Timothy Wilson (2004), is that most information processing resides outside of consciousness for functional reasons (efficiency) rather than emotional reasons (repression).

2.1 Strangers We Already Know

As the father of psychotherapy, Freud (1912) made *transference* the centerpiece of his procedural approach. Simply put, transference is said to occur when past experiences with others become confounded with subsequent relationships. Freud, along with many others, believed that transference is unconscious and automatic. The long-standing clinical tradition in psychotherapy has been to evoke these unconscious misattributions so that they can be consciously identified and corrected.

As suggested by the psychodynamic tradition, research by Morsella (2005) has found that achieving awareness of an implicit mental process can provide a basis for controlling it. However, in contrast to Freud, cognitive scientists now believe that all emotional reactions to others involve unconscious perception and memory. In other words, *transference is not pathological.*

These entanglements of the past and the present are part of everyday social encounters and are most likely to occur in response to new people. The concept of *entangled selves* has been proposed by Andersen and Chen (2002) to show how unique aspects of one's personality emerge whenever we come into contact with another person who serves as an unconscious prime to the relationship with a past significant other.

People automatically come to like or dislike other people they meet by virtue of some minimal resemblance he or she has to a significant other. Rather than using the term *transference*, researchers speak of "significant-other representations." In keeping with clinical theory, modern researchers have found that rich and complex representations of a significant other can affect a whole array of responses to a stranger who resembles that significant other.

For example, if the overall feeling experienced in childhood with your sister, Tracy, was negative and conflictual, then the woman at work who is also named Tracy and has the same color of hair may find herself frequently catching your ire. Even more interestingly, your behavior is likely to be less mature, because it is a younger personality that has been primed. In other words, transference responses range from mood, to impressions, to expectations as well as interpersonal behavior. Andersen and Berenson (2001) have shown in laboratory tests that these effects occur without any awareness that the representation from the past affects current responses to the stranger.

Thus, when this activation of implicit memory occurs, the person experiencing the emotional and behavioral effects (transference reaction) is unlikely to recognize these associations. Additionally, there may be content memories and specific triggers that remain outside of conscious awareness.

This brings us back to the example at the opening of the chapter—a woman who had possibly been abused by a priest was triggered by symbols of priestly power.

Another important finding by James Uleman and colleagues (2004) is that when the strength of explicit impressions is compared to implicit impressions, unconscious associations produce the most enduring effects. This would help explain why transference reactions are so difficult to revise. No matter how much you smile and say kind things, that one person in the crowd may still despise you or, conversely, may feel love at first sight.

When gifted therapists, such as Aaron Beck or Milton Erickson, encounter transference reactions, rather than making a transference interpretation, they take an empathetic stance—endeavoring to better understand the person's experience. Accordingly, researchers such as Piper and colleagues (1991) have found an inverse relationship between transference interpretations and therapy outcomes. For those seeking to protect the therapeutic alliance, there is an overt attempt to support the client and help him find words to express his needs, whether they be hostile, romantic, or peculiar. After the client feels acknowledged or understood, my approach is to move the focus of attention away from myself by asking, "Was there another time you felt this same way? If so, what was happening?" The first reply is typically, "I can't think of anything right now." My next suggestion is that if my client will wait just a moment and focus on the general feeling, he might be surprised by what suddenly comes to memory (conscious process work). A similar recall technique was described many years ago by Prince (1912), who wrote:

> A person may remember any given experience in a general way, such as what he does during the course of the day, but the minute details of the day he ordinarily forgets. Now, if he allows himself to fall into a passive state of abstraction, simply concentrating his attention upon a particular past moment, and gives free reign to all the associative memories belonging to that moment that float into his mind, at the same time taking care to forgo all critical reflection upon them, it will be found that the number of details that will be recalled will be enormously greater than can be recovered by voluntary memory. Memories of the details of each successive moment follow one another in continuous succession.
>
> (24–25)

Moving way beyond Freudian theory, researchers have also found that our social reactions are influenced by implicit memories of interactions with the individual in front of us. This dynamic was illustrated in a clever film, *50 First Dates*, in which anterograde amnesia prevents a woman from retaining new explicit memories, though the influence of implicit memories remains intact. As suggested by the filmmakers, it is possible to experience an implicit memory that produces feelings and intuitions that come from past encounters with a particular person, but which we are unable to consciously recall.

For example, Levinson (1965) described an interesting response from a woman who came out of surgery inexplicably weepy, depressed, and aversive to her surgeon. The reasons for her reaction were unclear until Levinson, on a hunch, hypnotized the woman and regressed her to the time of the surgery. During this exploration, the woman blurted out, "The surgeon says it might be malignant!" Further inquiry revealed that the doctors had discovered a possible malignancy during the surgery and had discussed it while she was anesthetized. Apparently, unconscious perception during anesthesia can result in implicit processing paired with conscious emotional states. This is one of two basic ways in which the emotional unconscious can be expressed (the emotion is conscious, but the source of that emotion remains unconscious).

2.2 Hybrid Reactions

When I speak of hybrid reactions, I am referring to processing that is taking place on two levels—conscious and unconscious. Recall the example above of the woman becoming infuriated at me without understanding why. This type of reaction is known to researchers as sudden emotionality, and it demonstrates how perception can operate at strictly unconscious levels and still activate conscious emotional states. Let's consider a straightforward example that does not involve theoretical defense mechanisms.

On this occasion, two women had panic attacks on the same day at the exact same moment. One of the women contacted her psychiatrist to report intense feelings of anxiety, fear of falling, heart palpitations, and depersonalization. While in this state of panic, she hid under her bed. Shortly after, she received a call from her friend, who had just had her worst panic attack in years—at precisely the same time of day.

After some investigation, it was discovered that an earthquake, registering magnitude six on the Richter scale, had occurred at exactly the time of the two patients' panic episodes. Neither woman had conscious knowledge of the earth tremor because it was too weak to be consciously felt (Traub-Werner 1989). While their emotional reactions were able to emerge into conscious awareness, the perception of the tremor remained subliminal.

As illustrated in the earthquake example, researchers, such as Winkielman and Berridge (2004), have found that emotions can be activated with subliminal stimuli and influence the actions of the individual without the person being aware of this influence.

In addition to emotional reactions to the unconscious perception of frightening events, research has shown that people also experience sudden emotionality in response to unconscious memories that have been triggered. Furthermore, it has been found that emotional responsiveness to unconsciously perceived information is much greater than consciously perceived information. In other words, implicit perception does not let things go.

This same dynamic (sudden emotionality with implicit memory) seems to be what Freud and Breuer (1895) had in mind in *Studies in Hysteria* when they wrote:

> Hysterics suffer mainly from reminiscences. [But in] the great majority of cases it is not possible to establish the point of origin by a simple interrogation of the patient, however thoroughly it may be carried out … principally because he is genuinely unable to recollect it and often has no suspicion of the causal connection between the precipitating event and the pathological phenomenon.
>
> (7)

While it would be a mistake to make this single unconscious dynamic a target of the entire therapeutic endeavor, as Freud did, it would also be naïve to dismiss the possibility of sudden emotionality without conscious recall for the causal connections.

2.3 Unconscious Emotion

The second way in which unconscious perceptions can be influential is when the triggered emotion is denied conscious representation. This has been described within the psychodynamic literature in terms of the classic Freudian defense mechanisms. Sigmund Freud (1923) described many defense mechanisms in his paper "The Ego and the Id," which were then extended in a paper by his daughter, Anna Freud (1936). These unconscious mechanisms are all assumed to block painful or repressed feelings and ideas from conscious awareness. The list of unconscious defenses includes: reaction formation (when a person behaves in a way opposite to the way he or she feels), displacement (when strong feelings triggered by one person are shifted onto another), intellectualization (when thinking is used to avoid feeling), and denial (blocking external events from awareness). The theoretical function of each of these is to render the person unaware of his or her deepest emotions.

While clinicians have over a century of experience working with unconscious emotions and motivations in distressed individuals, researchers have now shown that healthy individuals are also motivated by emotions they do not recognize. New developments in cognitive psychology make it apparent that the separation of emotion from conscious awareness occurs daily as a result of ordinary learning.

Given the perceptual limitations of conscious awareness, much of our learning involves the unconscious association of mental representations with emotional states. Given the neurological structure of the brain, it seems that there are forms of associative learning that are mediated by different neural structures from those involved in consciousness. In other words, we are unaware of many of our emotional reactions to stimuli simply because the associative processes that link affects and representations do not require consciousness.

The implication is that our emotional reactions may naturally form into multiple layers, some conscious and some unconscious. From my experience, unconscious emotion does not always interfere with conscious emotionality, but rather it adds an additional layer of understanding.

For example, wanting to test the clinical utility of a rating scale that measures emotions, I invited dozens of individuals to rate all of their emotional experiences from the previous week. Curiously, jealousy was never admitted. Even more curiously, when I interviewed the individuals, many appeared to be angry at another individual who was receiving benefits that they believed they deserved. When asked, their anger was conscious. But the "wanting" feelings of jealously did not emerge until more of their life story was explored. This led me to assume that jealousy is often experienced without conscious awareness.

In contrast, some people do not permit themselves to feel anger. These individuals are often labeled passive-aggressive, which is a lack of awareness of the anger that motivates a predictable pattern of hostile interaction.

Similarly, cardiology clinics frequently encounter patients who complain of behavioral and physiological symptoms associated with panic disorder, but they do not report feeling fear or distress. The patients typically report concern only about the symptoms themselves (Kushner and Beitman, 1990; Beitman et al., 1993). Just as with jealousy and anger, the experience of fear sometimes remains unconscious even as other emotions emerge.

After studying unconscious emotions in which the emotional quality of a stimulus is processed automatically, Phelps (2004) found that this automatic processing of emotion can influence attention and awareness. In other words, it is possible for unconscious perception to activate a strong fear reaction (my husband could die of heart failure), which leads to conscious avoidance of the subject matter. This can lead to bizarre scenarios, such as a woman wishing to plan a couple's ski trip with her husband for next winter, even as he lies in the hospital awaiting his third triple bypass surgery. This brings us to another influential Freudian concept—denial.

While repression is aimed at internal realities, denial, as defined by Freud (1924), is the refusal to acknowledge disturbing aspects of external reality. If the brain is biologically structured in such a way that a stimulus which evokes extreme fear can automatically trigger avoidance (diverting attention to something more amenable), it would help explain why defense mechanisms, such as repression and denial, occur.

In support of these clinical theories, cognitive neuroscience research suggests that the amygdala can detect the emotional properties of a stimulus prior to the signal reaching the prefrontal cortex, where explicit identification and awareness are formed. This neurologically based theory, known as LeDoux's system, argues that a disconnection between the amygdala and the cortex can produce a dissociation between explicit and implicit emotion.

LeDoux's system is intriguing because it suggests the presence of a memory function that operates independently of conscious working memory. This implicit memory system would permit the types of mental operations necessary for processing information outside of awareness and implementing unconscious choice. In the case of denial, emotion-laden information is diverted away from conscious awareness. But it is probably much more common for information (that has low emotional intensity) to be filtered from conscious review so as not to overwhelm a system with very limited perceptual capacity. The implication for therapy is that conscious processes are insufficient for accessing and coding implicit emotional information. That is why therapists need to use strategies designed to facilitate unconscious process work.

It is now widely accepted that emotions are an essential component in human problem solving. For example, Damasio (1999) argues that emotions automatically direct our attention toward more advantageous options, simplify decisions, and initiate rapid coping behavior, often before we are consciously aware that there is a problem. In the same way that respiration can increase or decrease without conscious recognition, it seems just as likely that emotions, in order to meet the demands of the immediate situation, could quickly rise and fall without requiring conscious processing.

Social psychology literature is replete with experimental data showing how people act on unconscious desires or fears or anger without having conscious emotional awareness. Everyday demonstrations of these phenomena are also abundant if you watch for them. For example, while in graduate school learning about a study on power and repressed anger, I saw a research video of a female graduate student being treated unfairly by a professor. She did not have sufficient social status to act on her anger, so the emotion seems to have been repressed. Throughout the professor's comments, the student sat quietly nodding in agreement. What was interesting was what happened with her hand as it rested casually over her knee. Her middle finger was extended and pointed towards the professor—a clear display of symbolized aggression. When interviewed, the student was shocked to see what her hand had done. Curious about what I had seen, I decided to pay more attention to people's fingers as they comply with situations they do not like. I have seen the behavior repeated on numerous occasions. Sometimes towards me, and once by a speaker on a panel sat before an audience of two hundred people. She apparently did not like the comments of another panelist (who was joking about encouraging his teenage son to experiment with dangerous street drugs).

Irrespective of the emotion that has been activated outside of conscious awareness, there is now experimental evidence suggesting that people can have subliminally triggered emotional reactions that drive judgment and behavior, even in the absence of any conscious feelings for these reactions (Winkielman and Berridge, 2004). Furthermore, under some conditions an emotional process may remain unconscious even when the person is attentive and motivated to describe his or her feelings correctly. As psychotherapists have long suspected, Winkielman and colleagues (2005) have now shown that even while remaining inaccessible to conscious awareness, this emotional process may nevertheless drive the person's behavior and physiological reactions.

What this means for therapy is that, on more occasions than not, clients will not be able to rely on conscious awareness to fully explain their reactions to events or significant people in their lives. Rather, clients are better equipped to provide a narrative of their ongoing interactions (though this is also subject to distortion). People can observe themselves in action much better than they can monitor their internal reactions. As the narrative is produced, clients' affective reactions reactivate and appear as micro-expressions (rapid displays of emotion). The therapist has the benefit of observing the facial expressions that accompany emotions as well as a behavioral sketch and personal narrative that imply hidden motives and unconscious attitudes.

2.4 Is Non-volitional Behavior Unconscious Will?

Having reviewed the surprising extent to which daily action is triggered by unconscious perception, we are forced to question the reality of conscious choice. Studies have suggested that after choice is triggered intention is constructed.

As an example, in a Fourneret and Jeannerod (1998) study participants were asked to trace a line displayed on a computer monitor while their hand was hidden by a mirror. However, the line that was displayed was not the same as the lines participants drew. Nevertheless, all expressed confidence that their hands had moved in the direction shown on the screen. In other words, these individuals had to rely on external feedback in order to construct their volitional will.

At this time, most researchers agree that two separate cortical visual pathways are activated during the perception of human movement: a dorsal one for action tendencies based on that information, and a ventral one used for the understanding and recognition of it (Decety and Grèzes, 1999; Rizzolatti et al., 1996). The psychological implication is that we may produce two different representations of the same object: one "pragmatic" and the other "semantic." The pragmatic representations are used for interacting with the object, while the semantic representation is for knowing about and identifying the object. Thus, the pragmatic representation (dorsal stream) could drive behavior in response to environmental stimuli in the absence of conscious awareness or understanding of that external information (Jeannerod, 2003; Farrer et al., 2003).

Other research by Perani and colleagues (1999) has shown that merely hearing action verbs (verbal representation) activates implicit motor representations. These verbs also activate working memory structures, such as the dorsolateral prefrontal cortex, the anterior cingulate, and premotor and parietal cortices.

These are the regions of the brain that are needed to carry out learned behavior in an uncertain environment. So if I say to a client, "You seem to be reaching out for help," a twitch in the client's hand, as if getting ready to reach forward, should not come as a surprise. The same happens if you move close to someone with your hand stretched out. An automatic movement will thrust their hand forward (for a handshake) before there is time to formulate conscious intention.

Accordingly, Jeannerod and Frak (1999) have found that mere observation of a meaningful action will activate the same brain area responsible for such movements. As it turns out, a large amount of human behavior is based on mimicry. It is not just that we cough when others cough or turn to face the same direction as others in the elevator. Most of the things we do and say are based to some extent on the imitation of those around us. Otherwise, there would be no such thing as culture, shared beliefs, or even language.

As argued by Bargh and Chartrand (1999), these are some of the environmental triggers of automatic behavior, which occurs without the necessity of the individual forming a conscious intention to behave that way, or without the individual knowing the true purpose of the behavior. If we want a given behavior to activate the feeling of volition, the movement needs to be preceded by approximately two seconds with a conscious representation of that action. This is enough time for the part of the brain that controls movement to establish a link with the part of the brain that makes meaning of movement. This post hoc connection occurs when we establish intention. But it does not mean our intention produced the movement.

While hypnosis has long made use of this neuro-structural characteristic (to generate expectancy effects), what modern research is showing, to a startling degree, is just how unaware we are of how we move and what causes these movements to occur. More specifically, recent neurological studies have established the dissociation between motoric behavior and conscious awareness as a basic structural feature of the human brain. While intended movements are normally represented in the prefrontal and premotor cortex, the representations used to guide action are in the parietal cortex.

Based on the body of research reviewed here, it seems that automatic movements produced during hypnosis are more directly represented in the parietal cortex, while bypassing the prefrontal cortex, thereby severing the link between conscious intention and movement. Furthermore, if the hypnotist states that an action will occur (such as eye closure), just before the action occurs (exploiting the blink reflex) volitional control will seem to transfer outside of the subject to the hypnotist (he made my eyes close).

Therefore, a hypnotherapist can tell a client to relax and make no intentional movements. But after saying something about a hand becoming lighter and then moving his hand upward ever so slightly, the client is shocked and amazed to see his own hand lift without intention (the automatic movement is primed verbally and visually through social mimicry). To explain this response, Erickson and colleagues (1976, 247–248) point out, "Most people do not know of their total capacities for response to stimuli. They place mystical meanings on much of the information they get by subtle cues."

From a biological perspective, Cojan and colleagues (2015) found differences in the activation of the parietal cortex and anterior cingulate regions of the brain when comparing high versus low hypnotizable subjects. This provides a clearer explanation for certain hypnotic phenomena. Rather than assuming mystical effects are produced by trance, we can acknowledge the normal limitations of conscious awareness and motoric functioning.

As we should now expect, the same behavior occurs outside the context of hypnosis. For example, because of my knowledge of embodied emotion, I can look at a client's movements and say with confidence, "That conversation you had with your son really touched your heart." With a look of surprise due to the emotional saliency of my wording, the client will respond, "Yes. How did you know?"

If I do not think she will feel overly exposed (shamed), I will explain, "As you began to tell me what he said to you, you placed your hand over your heart." Quickly, the client will look down to locate her hand and re-establish the neural link (between prefrontal cortex and parietal cortex) by intentionally moving her hand to her lap. My experience has been that this somatic reorientation is required whenever the initial movement was purely automatic.

Similarly, Peter Levine (1997) has built an entire system of trauma therapy (Somatic Experiencing) around this practice of reorienting to the body following a trauma. The reason this makes so much sense is because during a traumatic event there is a flood of automatic movements and a loss of intentionality. With PTSD there seems to be an enduring dissociation between the semantic and pragmatic regions of the brain. In order to re-establish the experience of volitional control, the link between movement and intention must be re-established.

This principle is best illustrated in cases involving movement disorders, which certainly undermine the feeling of having volitional control. On several occasions I have had children and adults seek help for movement disorders of the most extreme degree. One teenage boy had to be strapped into his bed at night because his convulsions were so severe that they threw him to the ground. Requiring a cane, he could barely walk and could not feed himself. As he sat on my couch, his arms flailed about wildly until I initiated hypnosis. After that he was perfectly still. The parents could not believe their eyes.

During hypnosis, he was no longer seeking to use conscious intention to control his movements. Instead, he became dependent on external primes (my use of touch and verbal suggestion). But as soon as the hypnosis ended, the problem returned. While in my office, the unintended movements were less severe, but meaningful progress outside the office was only achieved after months of seeking to re-establish a feeling of control over his life (not only for his body but also for events occurring within the family).

If you read about movement disorders in the hypnosis literature, you will find similar outcomes. The hypnotic miracle is temporary. It only lasts as long as the external guidance endures. More substantial gains come from teaching the client how to use indirect methods of motoric control. This is no different from teaching an emotionally unstable client how to use imagery, breathing techniques, or CBT as indirect controls of emotion.

When there is organic brain damage, the process of re-establishing volitional control takes months. Because the cognitive thoughts and the motor representations (used to guide behavior) are apparently held in anatomically separate parts of the brain, some patients with brain damage are no longer able to link their intentions to their actions. This occurs when there is impairment in the location where intended movements are represented but no impairment in the location where action systems operate (Frith and Frith, 2001). Due to neuroplasticity, this neural link can be re-established with the right type of practice.

Baumeister and Masicampo (2010) made the interesting argument that because of its severe limitations, the function of conscious will is not able to organize behavior for solving problems but rather to associate our actions with a feeling, thus allowing us to sense in a very basic way what type of person we are (identity formation).

Similarly, Clore (1992) argues that this feeling of personal agency or intent is an intuitive accounting system that makes us feel we deserve things—good or bad. Without this feeling, we would be deprived of the experience of personal emotions, such as pride and disappointment, thus there would be no comprehension of achievement. Nor would there be a moral sense created by principled emotions, such as guilt and obligation.

In the same way that feelings of purpose or joy or hope are important to our psychological survival, I would argue that *the feeling of volition is essential to mental health.* This feeling can either be diminished or embellished depending on the nature of the challenges we face and which system of intelligence we employ.

Paradoxically, for individuals to succeed in regulating how they physically interact with the surrounding environment, it seems that unconscious representation (non-volitional will) is best suited for the task. This dynamic is reflected in the common advice coaches give to their athletes, "Get out of your head and get your body into the game." In contrast, abstract intellectual tasks, such as solving a calculus problem, are the province of conscious effort (volitional will) and therefore best resolved with focused conscious attention.

2.5 Primes, Prediction, Suggestion, and Self-organizing Change

Things are not always as they appear, especially when it comes to conscious perception and self-determination. Following the lead of philosophy and science (providence of conscious effort), traditional forms of psychotherapy have attempted to use conscious reason to gain control over unconscious processes. The problem with that strategy is that conscious thought occurs too far downstream to change emotional reactions or to even preempt physical movement. For example, if you set your hand on something hot, the arm will jerk away long before you have time to think about initiating movement or even consciously experience the pain. Conscious thought is more like a splash, something that happens after the stone hits the water.

If our conscious intentions are so ill-equipped for managing explicit behavior and consciously processed emotions, it prompts the question, How should we ever hope to regulate unconscious processes?

One answer seems to be the use of priming to establish unconscious goals. A prime is essentially any stimulus that influences a person's near-term thoughts and actions (in contrast to suggestion, which aims to influence long-term thoughts and actions).

For the simplest illustration, think of the 18-year-old boy soldier sent to war in the early twentieth century. Far from home, sitting in a ditch trembling with fear, our **you**ng soldier **can** pull out a photograph of his mother or girlfriend and suddenly recompose himself, find a renewed sense of strength, and continue with his mission. The small item serves as a prime for an unconscious goal that is built into secure attachment relationships (stay alive for others). I **do** know more than one person who has clearly defied death for the sake of this implicit goal.

Given the evidence we have recently examined, there is reason to believe that unobtrusive primes (supraliminal yet unconscious) are the best choice for mediating implicit activity. **This** can include the use of symbols, gestures, written statements (with long exposure time), or verbalized concepts that are interspersed throughout ordinary conversation. As an example of the interspersal technique, I have placed a simple message above, using bold font (i.e., **you can do this**).

During speech, verbal primes are achieved by emphasizing single words, such as *hope* or *determination*, perhaps within the context of a story. This is just one step away from the use of indirect suggestion, which occurs when instructions for long-term behavior are hidden within the context of a story.

For example, while speaking to a suicidal young man in imminent danger (who had been savagely shamed as a child by his father), I made the off-hand remark, "Most of us struggle if we do not have a father to validate us, someone to look us in the eyes and say, '*You are a person of worth*!'" I used an indirect suggestion so that implicit processes could start to reorganize themselves around the idea rather than having short-lived conscious processes struggle with the task. Before departing, this person commented that he wanted to stay, because he felt safe in my office. So, I had him use his phone to take a selfie with me (a prime). I had him position his camera so that a second embedded prime was in the background—a framed picture that I will describe later.

For most of us, unobtrusive primes will be the easiest method for bypassing conscious awareness, thereby activating unconscious processes (without conscious oversight). If you are a gifted hypnotist, you can use suggestions in the same way, but not everyone can create the amnesic barrier needed to prevent conscious interference.

To be realistic, we should recognize that priming will not work in all circumstances, and its effects are limited. Merchants cannot subliminally flash a picture of Pepsi on a movie screen and expect everyone in the audience to stand up and go purchase a Pepsi. However, if someone had already decided to go grab a drink, the prime could influence which brand of soda suddenly came to mind.

As shown by Cartwright (1959), when priming succeeds, you can affect a person's behavior by making some motivations more salient than others. But you cannot give the person a motivation that he or she does not already have. Nor can you make the person do something for which he or she has no desire or interest. For priming to produce a meaningful effect, the primed behavior must be relevant and appropriate for the immediate situation in which people find themselves.

Rather than thinking of priming as a means of clandestine control, it is more accurate to think of priming as a path to existing mental representations. An effective prime merely makes certain relevant mental representations (e.g., memories, images, thoughts) more accessible and "within reach."

As an example, I can describe one of several unobtrusive primes used in my office. Wishing to evoke feelings of comfort and security as well as unconscious receptivity to caring behavior, I placed a picture in the office that depicts an act of loving support.

My prime is a commercial photo of a small boy who has fallen asleep on top of his father while visiting the beach. This poster-sized image is placed to the side of my chair. This is what is meant by unobtrusive prime—something easily seen but not necessarily noticed.

I chose this image after reading research in the attachment literature. Using images with loving interactions as a prime, Mikulincer and others (2001) were able to activate increased feelings of security, openness to support, and increased cognitive flexibility (openness to new ideas). These were behaviors that I believed would be beneficial to the therapeutic endeavor.

Curiously, most clients do not pay conscious attention to the image during the first few visits. However, after making progress in therapy and reconnecting with powerful emotional states, some clients will suddenly notice the picture. Typically, they ask, "Is that a new picture?" After I explain that it has been there all along, the next question is, "Is that a picture of you?"

Presumably, the caring and protective nature of the therapy setting activates feelings towards me as a father surrogate. If the client is identifying with the vulnerability of the child in the photo, the automatic perception would be that I am the father in the photo. As mentioned above, when I invited the client with suicidal urges to take a selfie with me, this was the picture that was in the background. As for outcomes, a few weeks later this client called to thank me. As he put it, "I would not be alive today if you hadn't been willing to see me" (the visit was during a holiday). He explained that after leaving my office, he contacted his father and told him for the first time about his suicidal urges. The father took him in immediately and paid for therapy/hospitalization in the state where he lived.

Because primes are short-lived (often no more than 48 hours), it is often useful to follow up with the use of prediction. For example, while working with a client who has suffered trauma, I might make an unobtrusive prediction,

"The safe, comfortable feeling that you have here in my office will probably stay with you, especially if your mind happens to flashback to this session."

For greater effect, I can use the weight of my authority to make an even stronger prediction. For example, "You have reached a certain milestone in your therapy. Given your current rate of progress, I have no doubt that it will soon become much easier for you to see kindness and consideration extended to you by others—something that has actually been there all along but that was obscured by the effects of trauma." Even though it sounds specific, the prediction is ambiguous, leaving space for self-organizing change.

It seems that positive predictions are extremely beneficial to unconscious processing. When done responsibly, positive prognostication helps activate a special type of motivation known as promotion focus. The prediction creates an unconscious fixation on a tangible reward (especially if the object is highly desired). This type of focus produces carryover effects. Specifically, Urry and colleagues (2004) found that personal-goal-directed approach motives (promotion focus) are associated with greater happiness and meaning in life.

An important point to recognize is that automatic activation can occur only if the individual has that behavioral representation available in the first place. In other words, the soldier mentioned earlier would not get much help from a photo of his mom if she had been an abusive and emotionally unavailable woman. When I have encountered individuals with such a childhood (perhaps physically tortured by both parents), I have successfully activated secure attachment reactions after using primes connected to real-life experience.

In one such instance, I was able to generate remarkable emotional shifts in a chronically violent individual by having him tell me about a day in his childhood that was spent with a big, affectionate, yellow dog (the only living creature he could recall that showed him love). His spontaneous reaction to this (self-generated) prime was to ask me if I thought it was possible that the woman he was living with might also love him. I replied with a prediction, "There is only one way to find out. If you show her love, she might decide to return it."

The effects of this brief intervention were profound. He decided on his own to write a poem (creative imagination) as a way of telling this woman that he loved her. Having grown up as an orphan in a Hell's Angels biker gang, she was hardened and had never had anyone say such a thing to her. This awkwardly read piece of poetry marked the end of the physical violence that had previously characterized their relationship.

The therapeutic use of prediction is a topic we will return to and explore in greater detail in Chapter 6.

Meanwhile, the point to be taken from this chapter is that conscious intention cannot rule our lives—its perceptual scope, depth, and processing capacity are far too limited. Imagine trying to drive a car on the highway while only peering into the rearview mirror (a post hoc resource). An overwhelming amount of research shows that while conducting day-to-day activities our actions are constantly influenced by unconscious stimuli that result in implicit memories, attitudes, learning, evaluations, and planning. As will be explained later, for those who indulge themselves in creative imagination, there is also implicit choice (non-volitional will). This is not to say conscious intention has zero value; rather, its function is best utilized in combination with a strong appeal to an unconscious intelligence—the central aim of unconscious process work.

Chapter 2 Key Points

- Our perception of others is almost always shaped by unconscious memories of another person who bears a resemblance or filled a similar role (transference). This primes the same automatic behavior that was learned in the prior relationship.
- Our perception of our mind's inner workings (e.g., emotion, intention, and choice) is based on observations of our external actions and automatic guesswork.
- People can have emotional reactions that remain inaccessible to conscious awareness while driving that person's behavior and physiological reactions.
- While ideas about conscious intent help shape our identity, actual self-regulation is best achieved by unconscious processes.
- Priming is the easiest way to reduce conscious interference while activating unconscious problem-solving processes.

References

Andersen, Susan, and Kathy R. Berenson. 2001. "Perceiving, Feeling, and Wanting: Motivation and Affect Deriving from Significant-Other Representations and Transference." In *The Social Mind: Cognitive and Motivational Aspects of Interpersonal Behavior*, edited by J. P. Forgas, K. D. Williams, and L. Wheeler, 231–256. Cambridge: Cambridge University Press.

Andersen, Susan M., and Serena Chen. 2002. "The Relational Self: An Interpersonal Social-Cognitive Theory." *Psychological Review* 109 (4): 619–645. doi:10.1037/0033-295X.109.4.619.

Bargh, John A., and Tanya L. Chartrand. 1999. "The Unbearable Automaticity of Being." *American Psychologist* 54 (7): 462–479. doi:10.1037/0003-066X.54.7.462.

Baumeister, Roy F., and E. J. Masicampo. 2010. "Conscious Thought Is for Facilitating Social and Cultural Interactions: How Mental Simulations Serve the Animal-Culture Interface." *Psychological Review* 117 (3): 945–971. doi:10.1037/a0019393.

Beitman, Bernard D., Vaskar Mukerji, Johnna L. Russell, and Melanie Grafing. 1993. "Panic Disorder in Cardiology Patients: A Review of the Missouri Panic/Cardiology Project." *Journal of Psychiatric Research* 27 (1): 35–46. doi:10.1016/0022-3956(93)90016-U.

Cartwright, Dorwin, ed. 1959. *Studies in Social Power*. Ann Arbor, MI: University of Michigan.

Clore, Gerald L. 1992. "Cognitive Phenomenology: Feelings and the Construction of Judgment." In *The Construction of Social Judgments*, edited by Leonard L. Martin and Abraham Tesser, 133–164. New York: Psychology Press.

Cojan, Yann, Camille Piguet, and Patrik Vuilleumier. 2015. "What Makes Your Brain Suggestible?: Hypnotizability Is Associated with Differential Brain Activity during Attention Outside Hypnosis." *NeuroImage* 117: 367–374. doi:10.1016/j.neuroimage.2015.05.076.

Damasio, Antonio R. 1999. *The Feeling of What Happens: Body and Emotion in the Making of Consciousness.* New York: Houghton Mifflin Harcourt.

Decety, Jean, and Julie Grèzes. 1999. "Neural Mechanisms Subserving the Perception of Human Actions." *Trends in Cognitive Sciences* 3 (5): 172–178. doi:10.1016/S1364-6613(99)01312–01311.

Erickson, Milton H., Ernest L. Rossi, and Sheila I. Rossi. 1976. "Hypnotic Realities: The Induction of Clinical Hypnosis and Forms of Indirect Suggestion." In *Hypnotic Realities: The Induction of Clinical Hypnosis and Forms of Indirect Suggestion*, Vol. 10. Phoenix, AZ: Milton H. Erickson Foundation Press.

Farrer, C., N. Franck, N. Georgieff, C. D. Frith, J. Decety, and M. Jeannerod. 2003. "Modulating the Experience of Agency: A Positron Emission Tomography Study." *NeuroImage* 18 (2): 324–333. doi:10.1016/S1053-8119(02)00041–00041.

Fourneret, Pierre, and Marc Jeannerod. 1998. "Limited Conscious Monitoring of Motor Performance in Normal Subjects." *Neuropsychologia* 36 (11): 1133–1140. doi:10.1016/S0028-3932(98)00006–00002.

Freud, Anna. 1936. *Das Ich Und Die Abwehrmechanismen* [*The Ego and the Defense Mechanisms*]. Oxford: Internationaler Psychoanalytischer Verlag.

Freud, Sigmund. (1912) 1959. "The Dynamics of the Transference." In *Sigmund Freud Collected Papers*, edited by James Strachey, translated by Joan Riviere, Vol. 2, 312–322. New York: Basic Books.

Freud, Sigmund. (1923) 2018. "The Ego And The Id (1923)." *TACD Journal* 17 (1): 5–22. doi:10.1080/1046171X.1989.12034344.

Freud, Sigmund. 1924. "The Loss of Reality in Neurosis and Psychosis." In *The Standard Edition of the Complete Psychological Works of Sigmund Freud*, 19, edited by James Strachey, 183–187. London: Hogarth Press. https://www.pep-web.org/document.php?id=se.021.0001a#p0003.

Freud, Sigmund, and Joseph Breuer. (1895) 2004. *Studies in Hysteria.* New York: Penguin.

Frith, Uta, and Chris Frith. 2001. "The Biological Basis of Social Interaction." *Current Directions in Psychological Science* 10 (5): 151–155. doi:10.1111/1467-8721.00137.

Jeannerod, Marc. 2003. "The Mechanism of Self-Recognition in Humans." *Behavioural Brain Research* 142 (1): 1–15. doi:10.1016/S0166-4328(02)00384–00384.

Jeannerod, Marc, and Victor Frak. 1999. "Mental Imaging of Motor Activity in Humans." *Current Opinion in Neurobiology* 9 (6): 735–739. doi:10.1016/S0959-4388(99)00038–0.

Kihlstrom, John F. 2013. "Chapter 12: Unconscious Processes." In *The Oxford Handbook of Cognitive Psychology*, edited by Daniel Reisberg, 176–186. New York: OUP USA.

Kushner, Matt G., and Bernard D. Beitman. 1990. "Panic Attacks without Fear: An Overview." *Behaviour Research and Therapy* 28 (6): 469–479. doi:10.1016/0005-7967(90)90133–90134.

Levine, Peter. 1997. *Waking the Tiger: Healing Trauma: The Innate Capacity to Transform Overwhelming Experiences.* New York: North Atlantic Books. https://www.secondsale.com/i/waking-the-tiger-healing-trauma-the-innate-capacity-to-transform-overwhelming-experiences/9781556432330?gclid=EAIaIQobChMInd2PtNKJ6wIVrD6tBh3WMQTQEAYYAiABEgLodfD_BwE.

Levinson, Harry. 1965. "The Future of Health in Industry." *Industrial Medicine & Surgery* 34 (April): 321–334.

Mikulincer, Mario, Gilad Hirschberger, Orit Nachmias, and Omri Gillath. 2001. "The Affective Component of the Secure Base Schema: Affective Priming with Representations of Attachment Security." *Journal of Personality and Social Psychology* 81 (2): 305–321. doi:10.1037/0022-3514.81.2.305.

Morsella, Ezequiel. 2005. "The Function of Phenomenal States: Supramodular Interaction Theory." *Psychological Review* 112 (4): 1000–1021. doi:10.1037/0033-295X.112.4.1000.

Perani, Daniela, Stefano F. Cappa, Tatiana Schnur, Marco Tettamanti, Simona Collina, Màrio Miguel Rosa, and Ferruccio Fazio. 1999. "The Neural Correlates of Verb and Noun Processing: A PET Study." *Brain* 122 (12): 2337–2344. doi:10.1093/brain/122.12.2337.

Phelps, Elizabeth A. 2004. "The Interaction of Emotion and Cognition: The Relation Between the Human Amygdala and Cognitive Awareness." In *The New Unconscious*, edited by Ran R. Hassin, James S. Uleman, and John A. Bargh, 61–76. Oxford: Oxford University Press.

Piper, William E., Hassan F. A. Azim, Anthony S. Joyce, and Mary McCallum. 1991. "Transference Interpretations, Therapeutic Alliance, and Outcome in Short-Term Individual Psychotherapy." *Archives of General Psychiatry* 48 (10): 946–953. doi:10.1001/archpsyc.1991.01810340078010.

Prince, Morton. 1912. *The Unconscious: The Fundamentals of Human Personality Normal and Abnormal*. New York: Macmillan.

Rizzolatti, G., L. Fadiga, M. Matelli, V. Bettinardi, E. Paulesu, D. Perani, and F. Fazio. 1996. "Localization of Grasp Representations in Humans by PET: 1. Observation versus Execution." *Experimental Brain Research* 111 (2): 246–252. doi:10.1007/BF00227301.

Traub-Werner, Daniel. 1989. "Anxiety in a Patient during an Unconsciously Experienced Earth Tremor." *The American Journal of Psychiatry* 146 (5): 679–680. doi:10.1176/ajp.146.5.679a.

Uleman, James S., Steven L. Blader, and Alexander Todorov. 2004. "Implicit Impressions." In *The New Unconscious*, edited by Ran R. Hassin, James S. Uleman, and John A. Bargh, 362–392. Oxford: Oxford University Press.

Urry, Heather L., Jack B. Nitschke, Isa Dolski, Daren C. Jackson, Kim M. Dalton, Corrina J. Mueller, Melissa A. Rosenkranz, Carol D. Ryff, Burton H. Singer, and Richard J. Davidson. 2004. "Making a Life Worth Living: Neural Correlates of Well-Being." *Psychological Science* 15 (6): 367–372. doi:10.1111/j.0956-7976.2004.00686.x.

Vermeule, Blakey. 2015. "The New Unconscious: A Literary Guided Tour." In *The Oxford Handbook of Cognitive Literary Studies*, edited by Lisa Zunshine, 463–482. New York: Oxford University Press. doi:10.1093/oxfordhb/9780199978069.013.0023.

Westen, Drew. 1999. "The Scientific Status of Unconscious Processes: Is Freud Really Dead?" *Journal of the American Psychoanalytic Association* 47 (4): 1061–1106. doi:10.1177/000306519904700404.

Wilson, Timothy D. 2004. *Strangers to Ourselves*. Cambridge, MA: Harvard University Press.

Winkielman, Piotr, and Kent C. Berridge. 2004. "Unconscious Emotion." *Current Directions in Psychological Science* 13 (3): 120–123. doi:10.1111/j.0963-7214.2004.00288.x.

Winkielman, Piotr, Kent C. Berridge, and Julia L. Wilbarger. 2005. "Unconscious Affective Reactions to Masked Happy Versus Angry Faces Influence Consumption Behavior and Judgments of Value." *Personality and Social Psychology Bulletin* 31 (1): 121–135. doi:10.1177/0146167204271309.

3 Choice and Deliberation

In this chapter, we will examine the domain of reason, which includes higher cognitive abilities, such as goal-setting, weighted choices, adaptive learning, and self-monitoring. Soon we will see that none of these processes are limited to conscious awareness. On the contrary, choice and deliberative thought involve both conscious and unconscious qualities.

As in the previous chapter, we will begin with familiar concepts and gradually expand our understanding, entering new territory that at first seems strange or impossible. While addressing the topic of unconscious self-determination, it is useful to start with the idea of rationalization.

In 1908, Ernest Jones introduced the term *rationalization* to the psychoanalytic literature. He defined this behavior as "the inventing of a reason for an attitude or action the motive of which is not recognized" (Jones, 1908, 163). The function of the behavior was assumed to be the defense of the ego. As Jones (1908, 163) explained, "No one will admit that he ever deliberately performed an irrational act, and any act that might appear so is immediately justified by … providing a false explanation that has a plausible ring of rationality." Thus, the key to rationalization was that the explanation (though false) seems logical. As with other defense mechanisms, we will soon see that the concept of rationalization has strong merit. The question to ask is whether rationalization is dysfunctional or normal everyday behavior.

With this question in mind, let us consider a study by Adrian North and colleagues (1999) on the role of implicit processing in reasoned evaluations. This field study examined consumers' awareness of why they chose one type of wine over another. As predicted, on certain days consumers purchased mostly German wine, and on other days they purchased mostly French wine. When asked about their choices, everyone had a rational explanation (e.g., a recent trip to Europe, tomorrow night's meal, etc.). But after two weeks, when asked again not a single person identified the actual cause of their behavior.

The controlled causal element was the music playing in the background. French music led to French wines outselling German ones, whereas German music contributed to consumers choosing German wines. This study, along with numerous others like it, led researchers to conclude that seemingly irrelevant situational cues can have a substantial impact on evaluations and

DOI: 10.4324/9781003127208-3

behavior. This is what is meant by *priming* (a strategic use of situational cues outside of conscious awareness).

3.1 Rationalization and Emotional Decision-Making

To make sense of this, it is helpful to go back 300 years to one of Europe's most important philosophers, David Hume (1711–1776). Due to what we recognize today as self-confirming biases, Hume argued that the only way to improve philosophy was to make the investigation of human nature empirical. In this regard, he anticipated the development of contemporary psychology. But, even more important for modern cognitive science was Hume's argument that conscious reasoning operates independently, without much need for contact with forces outside of itself. This led Hume to the conclusion that conscious awareness is not designed for working with complete causal explanations. As Hume (1800, 31) puts it, "These ultimate springs and principles are totally shut up from human curiosity and inquiry." In other words, we do what we do without really knowing why.

In a classic paper from 1977, Richard Nisbett and Timothy Wilson posed the question: To what extent are people aware of and able to report on the true causes of their behavior? The answer was not very well. While people firmly believe that they know their own minds, their reasons for behaving or choosing can be easily manipulated, often without their awareness.

For example, Nisbett and Wilson (1977) presented participants with an array of stockings as if they were in a consumer study and asked them to select their preference. Participants overwhelmingly chose the rightmost pair despite all pairs being identical. When asked the reason for their choice, participants did not mention the position of the stockings. When asked directly about the possibility of a position effect, participants denied it and felt either that they had misunderstood the question or were dealing with "a madman" (Nisbett and Wilson, 1977, 244).

Numerous studies since have shown that adults reconstruct their explanations for their own past behavior based on what seems to be the best fit for the actions that occurred. Introspection does not produce reliable results because the springs and principles are encapsulated in a windowless box.

Earlier, Daryl Bem (1965) produced evidence that an individual's best guess at why others have acted in a certain manner is no less accurate than insights about the individual's own personal actions. In both cases, people depend on observable evidence.

Bem's self-perception theory was initially intended to explain *cognitive dissonance*. A common example is known as the "spreading of alternatives," which occurs when subjects are forced to choose between two good alternatives. People subsequently rate the chosen alternative as the best choice and devalue the unchosen option. Any therapist who has worked with couples has undoubtedly seen this occur in the consulting room.

For example, when I have a couple that is in severe marital distress, and the husband tells his wife, "I never really loved you," my next question to the husband is, "How long have you been having an affair?" Though the accusation is sometimes denied, follow up information always yields the same results—he was cheating and subsequently lying to the therapist.

Even without the giveaway statement, when you observe an interaction pattern of one partner trying to save the marriage and the other devaluing this individual (who is clearly a kind, healthy, and dedicated spouse), then it is not a large leap of inference to hypothesize that the first partner has suddenly become faced with two compelling options—when only one can be openly embraced.

If you ask the partner why he or she chose to have the affair, the reasons are usually ego defensive. For example, "I endured a loveless marriage for as long as I could. I mentioned more than once that things had to improve, but she never seemed to listen."

In my thirty years of working with couples, never have I had an unfaithful partner respond:

> The detachment in our marriage began with my prioritization of work and internet pornography. My wife was constantly seeking a more intimate connection with me, but this felt exceedingly uncomfortable given that my mom was emotionally unavailable (from depression), and my father was also an unfaithful spouse who depended on narcissistic strategies rather than empathy to govern his relationships with others. In fact, I have strong narcissistic tendencies myself that make me emotionally unavailable and strain my ability to learn from my mistakes. Lastly, when I started going to bars after work and really enjoying myself there, I found my inhibitions against cheating sufficiently reduced that I was able to instigate an affair.

Reliable introspection does not seem to exist, neither inside nor outside the consulting room.

Returning to research, we will consider another remarkable study by Tanner and colleagues (2008). In this experiment, participants were provided with bowls of goldfish crackers and animal crackers. In one condition the participants predominantly chose to eat gold fish, and in the other they ate more animal crackers. When asked about their selections, participants explained that they had a special preference for the chosen item. What these individuals did not recognize was that they were mimicking the behavior of a confederate who was in the room eating either goldfish or animal crackers. The participants were not able to make this causal connection because there were no conscious thoughts about imitating someone else's eating behavior. Social mimicry is an automatic process.

The possibility that conscious preferences are invented after the fact (ad hoc constructions) and based on evidence of our behavior has been further substantiated by the phenomenon of *choice blindness*. Studies on this phenomenon show that people will not only confabulate reasons for arbitrary choices, but they will even generate explanations for a choice that they have *not made* (Johansson et al., 2014). We choose aesthetically pleasing explanations—not behaviors. But even this implicit choice is concealed from conscious awareness.

In studies on choice blindness, participants are asked to make choices (e.g., which of two faces is more attractive) and then to verbally explain their choice. What the participants do not know is that on some trials their choice has been replaced with the face they did not choose. Participants rarely notice that their selections have been reversed. Furthermore, they have no difficulty discussing the reasons for choices that they did not actually make—providing just as much detail and emotionality as for the non-manipulated choices. This apparent blindness extends to our most emotionally charged areas of choice, such as politics and moral decisions (Hall et al., 2012).

This same phenomenon seems to be what Shakespeare had in mind when he wrote *The Tragedy of Julius Caesar* (1599). The play opens with a crowd (normal society) being chastised for their change in loyalty from Pompey to Caesar (following Caesar's conquest), then their opinion turns against Caesar (after he is murdered), and then Mark Antony uses an emotional appeal to turn the crowd back against those who conspired against Caesar. All the while, the crowd remains blind to the reason for their fluid choices (follow those who currently hold power).

Due to the human need for consistency and meaning, awareness of a behavioral outcome leads people to attempt to understand why an outcome occurred (Why did I do that?). This need becomes particularly strong if an outcome is negative or unexpected, such as when an outcome conflicts with earlier choices or one's personal standards or social norms. This phenomenon is referred to in research as the *explanatory vacuum*, and it makes spontaneous confabulation more likely. As argued by Oettingen and colleagues (2006), when automatic behavior demands an explanation, a tendency to confabulate will appear. Commenting on this tendency, Dennett (1982, 173) writes, "It is not that they lie in the experimental situation, but that they confabulate; they make up likely sounding tales without realizing they are doing it; they … mistake theorizing for observing."

The same is true in therapy. When clients are asked to provide an explanation for unexpected behaviors, an explanation will be construed. These confabulations are genuinely believed and delivered with conviction. The story that is created can then have subsequent effects on the person's sense of self. As researchers have shown, once unexpected behavior is recognized, and a reason for the behavior is confabulated, this reason may become "sticky," leading to downstream effects in the form of new emotional reactions that drive subsequent behavior.

Similarly, Jonathan Haidt (2001) demonstrated that people's moral judgments are the result of emotional, fast, visceral reactions to social scenarios. When questioned, people will sometimes invent plausible-sounding rationales for their decisions, but experimental manipulation shows that these conscious intentions are constructed after the fact.

To better understand this, we can turn to the groundbreaking work of a neuroscientist, Antonio Damasio (1999), who treated patients suffering damage to the ventromedial prefrontal cortex. This is the area of the brain responsible for emotional processing, especially complex learned emotions. When damage to the brain spared the patients' rational faculties, Damasio observed that they had no trouble with memory, abstract reasoning, or math, and they performed well on IQ tests. However, these same patients could not make basic day-to-day decisions. Something as simple as choosing which cereal to eat became an impossible task. Apparently, without emotion, there is no way to establish preference or opinion, nor is it possible to evaluate the future consequences of one's actions. Damasio argued that these patients lack *somatic markers* (the experience of emotion within the body). This unconscious assignment of emotional values, which ordinarily accompanies our representations of the world, is also referred to as affect—the sensation of emotion.

Affect typically has an identifiable location within the body (somatic marker), which can be described with a variety of sensory qualities, such as tight, swirling, or empty. And like other somatic experiences, such as pain, affect can move in and out of conscious awareness. Thus, when we talk about having certain feelings, we are describing the experience of having affect come into conscious awareness (Basch, 1976). Damasio and his colleagues argue that our images or mental pictures of the world are imbued with the sensation of goodness or badness, urgency or lack of urgency—thus affect plays a crucial role in normal decision-making.

While conscious reason leads us to infer why we act as we do, emotion is what leads us to act. Given the imaging capabilities of modern neuroscience, evidence is mounting that conscious explanations come online rather late in the deliberative process—it takes a great deal of neuronal activity to crest into a signal that is supraliminal. Ever since Benjamin Libet's 1983 experiments showing how late that signal arrives, neuroscientists have debated what role consciousness plays in decision-making. Whatever influence it does wield seems to be rather indirect and slow to execute.

As stated earlier, the current consensus is that impulses to act begin in unconscious parts of the mind and may or may not pass through consciousness. While people sometimes mistakenly believe that their thoughts are responsible for actions, it is the instantaneous emotional reactions to external factors that reliably predict behavior. In contrast, conscious explanations more reliably predict a person's beliefs about how they should respond to a given situation and what constitutes socially acceptable behavior. Thus, verbal accounts of one's actions are typically a story, an exercise in rationalization.

The clear implication for psychotherapy is that any attempt to produce "true" introspective insight is naïve. Furthermore, the primary aim of cognitive behavioral therapy (CBT), which is to use cognition to transform emotion, may be equally misguided. As Leslie Greenberg (2012, 697) puts it, "Because much of the processing involved in the generation of emotional experience occurs independently of and prior to conscious thought, therapeutic work on a purely cognitive level of processing is unlikely to produce enduring emotional change." How much truer this must be when we consider the effect of unconscious emotion and unconscious primes.

3.2 Reverse Priming and Unconscious Choice

As you recall, Fredrick Myers was among the first to conceptually define unconscious processes and to speculate on their relevance to hypnosis, religion, and everyday experience. Myers believed that these operations were the result of a subliminal intelligence that possessed its own personality features, such as attitudes, beliefs, and moral convictions. As evidence of this invisible hand, Myers (1904) wrote,

> [Most] of us have observed that if we perform any small action to which there are objections, which we have once known but which have altogether passed from our minds, we are apt to perform it in a hesitating, inefficient way.
>
> (269)

Later, a similar principle would be discovered by John Ridley Stroop (1935), who created the Stroop Task (the first experimental procedure capable of measuring unconscious processes). To get a better understanding of the effect, read through the column of words below as quickly as possible, first reading the word silently and then saying out loud "big" if the font is big, "medium" if it is medium, or "small" if the font is small. GO!

BIG

small

MEDIUM

big

SMALL

For most people, there is a delay when speaking the final two words as compared with the first three. The latter require additional conscious effort to deal with the conflict between semantics and observation. We must force ourselves to say something that is apparently not true but still demanded. As Myers originally observed, we can only perform the behavior in a hesitating, inefficient way.

In studies of implicit racism, the same hesitation has been found for some individuals who do not consciously consider themselves racist, yet they hesitate when asked to pair a positive word with a person who is not included in their racial group (for a review see Dehon et al., 2017). These test outcomes turn out to be highly predictive of subsequent behavior (these individuals use racist behavior without realizing it).

Then, in 1999, Jack Glaser and Mahzarin Banaji made a fascinating discovery—when extreme subliminal primes are used (words with strong negative connotations) normal priming effects disappear. But, with moderate words they remain. For example, when subliminally primed with the word "dangerous" and then asked to pronounce correctly a word associated with black culture, the speed is likely quicker than with words associated with white culture if implicit racism is present. However, when the researchers used extreme primes, such as "Nazi" or "skinhead" (these words are more offensive than the word "dangerous"), the effect was reversed. Subjects made unconscious adjustments that were compensatory (they unconsciously sought to eliminate racial bias). This correction was achieved without consciously knowing what the prime was or how their behavior had changed! These researchers labeled this the *reverse priming effect*. In other words, the human mind can maintain unconscious vigilance over its own automatic processes and make corrections when something seems wrong (implicit self-regulation).

This degree of executive control would require an unconscious intelligence that can process the meaning of complex stimuli, arrange them categorically, and then evaluate them relative to established values or values that have been primed, such as "be accurate" or "be fair." These strategic yet unconscious compensations for unintended thoughts, feelings, or behaviors have been labeled by Glaser and Kihlstrom (2004) as *compensatory automaticity*.

Implicit self-regulation would not occur if unconscious processes were entirely passive (associative learning). Instead, it seems that there is an unconscious intelligence that has processing goals (e.g., accuracy, egalitarianism), which can operate independent of conscious intention. Furthermore, this intelligence is vigilant for threats to the attainment of these goals, and it will proactively compensate for such threats. In other words, *choice operates at multiple levels of consciousness*.

As Milton Erickson (1952) argued long ago, unconscious intelligence is capable of complex problem solving, automatic learning, and superior judgment. Subsequently, Erickson (1954; 1964) did not consider his use of indirect suggestion (unconscious goal activation) and behavioral directives (unconscious experiential learning) to be coercive but rather an appeal to unconscious will and self-organizing change (Erickson et al., 1976).

My experience as a clinician is that there is an implicit will that sometimes refuses to be violated. For example, while seeking to help a client become more emotionally self-aware (conscious process work), I helped him retrieve the following autobiographical narrative. At the time he was 52 years of age, and he stated that he had struggled since childhood with chronic depression, a poorly defined sense of self, volatile social connections, and no apparent goals (he moved frequently, never established himself professionally, and never married).

In contrast to these outcomes, he was exceptionally bright, he graduated with honors from an Ivy league college, he spoke multiple languages, and he could strike up a conversation with any stranger. These discrepancies led me to collect a more nuanced behavioral profile. I asked him to describe in minute detail pivotal moments in his adult life.

This request led him to reveal new facts, which he had omitted from earlier sessions. Most importantly, he recalled a passionate relationship with a woman from Canada, for whom he had great admiration and respect. Thinking that he might wish to marry her, he brought her to his hometown to meet his mother. During this meeting, the mother controlled the conversation and eventually decided to give some advice. Looking only at the girlfriend, she said, "You are going to have to take care of my son. He does not take care of himself so well." After that, my client could no longer stay in the relationship. He lost all interest and affection for this woman, whom he had been prepared to marry.

Curious, I asked if anything else like this had ever occurred. He then recalled another event when he was living in New York and working night and day to open a Sushi bar with a partner and friend. Both men were extremely hard-working. My client recognized that he had a strong passion and gift for food preparation. Right when they were ready to launch the restaurant, my client's mother decided that she wanted to meet his partner. During the conservation, she told this man, "You are going to have to take care of my son. He does not take care of himself so well." The next day, my client told his business partner he just couldn't do it. Soon after, he left New York and gave up on establishing himself as a professional chef. In contrast, his former partner went on to become a millionaire and a great success in the food industry.

If we use these behavioral outcomes to infer unconscious values, it seems safe to assume that some part of him was unwilling to be in a relationship where he would be dominated and controlled, which his mother had done throughout his childhood.

This conviction of will was apparently so strong that it prevented him from pursuing his conscious goals. Subsequently, he viewed these failures as evidence that he would never amount to anything in life—the sticky influence of a negative rationalization.

But if we trace his choices back to a pivotal moment, we see that his mother's comment(s) had an unconscious effect on how he framed his budding achievements. I believe the effect can best be described as a reverse prime. I say this because the words she used and the effect they achieved do not fit the description of verbal suggestion. Otherwise, he would have become excessively dependent on these individuals. Nor was it an instance of prediction (she did not predict his departure from the relationships). Her words merely served as a prime, making certain (intolerable) mental representations more accessible.

If we interpret his behaviors as an act of will, then we see that rather than merely hesitating (as happens in the lab), it became impossible for him to move forward with an action for which he had strong unconscious objections (entering a relationship based on dependency). As for follow up, at the time of this writing, my client had chosen to reconnect with his old friend, and he is now working with him doing commercial food preparation. I have advised him to avoid any contact with his mother until he is fully established in his new social identity. He agreed.

Not only has the unconscious capacity for an act of will been demonstrated experimentally, but it has also been shown that under the right conditions unconscious intelligence will compensate for anticipated threats to the attainment of its goals. This has led Glaser and Kihlstrom (2004) to argue that the unconscious is paradoxically "aware."

3.3 Implicit Experiential Learning

In one of the first books written on the subject of psychology in education, William James (1916) addresses the benefits of experience-based learning, which registers primarily as unconscious mental representations. As James (1916) states:

> Let no youth have any anxiety about the upshot of his education, whatever the line of it may be. If he keep faithfully busy each hour of the working day, he may safely leave the final result to itself. He can with perfect certainty count on waking up some fine morning to find himself one of the competent ones of his generation, in whatever pursuit he may have singled out. Silently, between all the details of his business, *the power of judging* in all that class of matter will have built itself up within him as a possession that will never pass away.
>
> (36)

The type of learning that James refers to is experientially based and primarily unconscious. This experiential learning results in the acquisition of new patterns of behavior in the absence of awareness of the patterns themselves.

James conceptualized this class of learning in terms of habit formation. However, modern research has revealed a more dynamic process. Research on implicit learning suggests that people learn all kinds of regularities about their environment, which become expressed in skilled performance even when they have no explicit knowledge of the complex covariations among social stimuli (if x and y, then q, but not for x alone). This decoding of rules means that implicit "grammars" are being used to generate inferences and actions (Lewicki, 1986; Rubin et al., 1993).

In contrast to arguments made by dual process theorists, such as Sigmund Freud and more recently Daniel Kahneman, substantial evidence now exists that unconscious intelligence can be as flexible, complex, controlling, deliberative, and action-oriented as conscious awareness. Bargh and Morsella (2008) also argue that this includes a capacity for highly-flexible, tentative adjustments during implicit learning. Using a variety of experimental manipulations, researchers have been able to teach new skills without the subject's awareness of the new ability. These conditions go far beyond the Pavlovian conditioning that automatically pairs a stimulus and a response. Rather, subjects are taught new complex behaviors that continue to evolve without conscious awareness.

In a lab setting, this is achieved by having the subject's conscious resources overloaded with separate tasks that consume working memory, such as counting backwards from 100 by threes. In a clinical setting, similar effects are achieved by focusing conscious attention on relaxing the body as unconscious intelligence evaluates new information. Or, the client might be told a compelling story so that (virtual) experiential learning occurs. Even better, the client will sometimes tell the therapist a story from her life that has embedded within it much of the learning needed to creatively address the current problem (the story's relevance is felt long before it is consciously understood). After the story is told to the therapist, all that is needed is explicit permission for the client to access this learning. For example, the therapist might say, "Wow, you were really resourceful at *that* time!" This both validates the skill set and acts as a prime to utilize the same resourceful behavior for the current problem.

The product of unconscious learning is intuition. When a person says to you, "I don't know why I know to do this, but I am confident this is what I must do," they are preparing to act on knowledge that has been acquired through unconscious learning. Thus, I use the term *intuition* as shorthand for unconscious causal reasoning and identification of solutions or goals.

The argument has been made that this helps explain the relative success of speed dating (intuitive evaluations) versus traditional dating (slow, deliberative evaluations). As most veteran therapists already know, just one glance into the client's eyes produces a readiness to act in a particular direction that later seems very appropriate for the client's mood, mindset, and even unstated goals. This flash of intuition is produced by years of implicit learning.

This brings us to the concept of premonition, which is a lay term that might also be connected to unconscious perception and learning. When pattern detection occurs at unconscious levels and learning occurs, an individual can develop an ability to accurately predict events in a way that defies conscious understanding. When tested in the laboratory, researchers found that subjects can acquire the ability to predict forthcoming events without being able to specify the underlying sequential structure, which they obviously learned (Lewicki et al., 1987). While people may sometimes mistake coincidence for premonition, those who are consistently accurate in their forecasts (without conscious understanding of that knowledge) may have the benefit of an exceptionally high unconscious intelligence.

When we talk about intuition or premonition, the implication is that we have acquired conscious knowledge of our insight. Thus, it is a hybrid reaction—conscious and unconscious processes are involved. However, this capacity for learning, prediction, and even goal setting can remain entirely unconscious. In these instances, the insights influence behavior without a corresponding intention and without awareness. During normal development, children learn a great deal from their families and social networks without conscious knowledge of the rules they have learned or how they continue to influence their actions. If these actions, which are unintentional and often occur outside of awareness, are not adaptive, then help might be indicated.

Therapists in general now recognize that for new rules to be learned at unconscious levels, experiential exercises are needed. Talk alone is not enough. Interestingly, research by Bowers and colleagues (1995) has shown that when people are given a challenging task, and they are able to achieve the correct solution, this implicit learning will continue to influence future behavior even though the individual is not consciously aware of the solution itself.

Lewicki, Hill, and Czyzewska (1992) have shown that people have no conscious access to the high-level processes needed for playing chess, feeling love, forming impressions of people, or problem solving and creative thinking. When asked how such judgments or decisions are generated, the subjects in these studies are unable to say how they knew what to do; all they know is that they "just do it." When we apply this to psychotherapy, with a lifetime of implicit learning, clients should be encouraged to trust what they know even without knowing how they know it.

3.4 A Psychic Whole

If we limit our understanding of unconscious processes to familiar Freudian defense mechanisms, it paints a picture of two independent systems—a segregationist, dualistic perspective that has information moving along two separate tracks. But the workings of the mind are more often integrated and mutually dependent. The same functionality should be expected during therapy. As argued by Morton Prince (1912) over 100 years ago, the conscious and unconscious form a psychic whole.

The contemporary theory that comes closest to arguing this same point is known as *cross-talk theory* (Baumeister and Masicampo, 2010). In contrast to dualistic theories, cross-talk argues that both types of consciousness enable different parts of the brain to share information (also known as global workspace theory)(Baars, 2005). Just as it is useful to have two eyeballs working together for the sake of depth perception, it seems that conscious and unconscious functions work together to achieve greater dimensionality.

For example, it has been found that unconscious dialogue (implicit self-talk) leads to decisions being made and the selection of goals. These capabilities then become integrated within the work of conscious processing as multiple systems work together. The implication for psychotherapy is that our methodology should be inclusive, fluidly moving between conscious and unconscious levels of awareness.

This contrasts with the disjointed clinical tradition of putting someone in a trance to access unconscious processes and then "waking them" to engage in conscious thought. Rather than breaking up therapeutic dialogue into a trance/non-trance staccato, unconscious process work can fluidly engage a psychic whole. The type of language most likely to promote cross-talk, which simultaneously stimulates multiple levels of awareness, will be explored in detail in Chapter 5.

3.5 Mental Segregation versus Utilization

In the same way that anthropologists learned to avoid ethnocentrism (using one's own value systems to judge others), I think we should be extraordinarily cautious when using conscious logic to judge unconscious choices. Condemnation instinctually leads to segregation. The more segregated the mental field becomes, the less likely an individual is to benefit from an integration of diverse abilities found at differing levels of consciousness. This is why it is so important to encourage clients to utilize their unconscious learning (intuitions and gut feelings). Just as importantly, we want clients to trust their critical thinking skills (probabilistic reasoning and hypothesis testing). But mental inclusiveness is not always easy.

Just as dream logic sometimes defies conscious understanding, the conclusions of unconscious learning sometimes seem a little bizarre or overblown. Subsequently, in the absence of understanding, we experience fear or aversion. This is illustrated in the following case report.

This case was described by Moshé Feldenkrais (1981), a Ukrainian-Israeli engineer and physicist and founder of the Feldenkrais Method (a system of physical exercise that seeks to increase self-awareness through movement). Though he was not trained as a psychotherapist, his study of movement disorders (created by injury) gave him a profound appreciation for implicit learning and unconscious goals.

His client was a woman in her sixties who complained of persistent acute pain in her lower abdomen above her pubis. Seeking help, she went to her GP, who ordered X-rays, blood, and urine analysis. Without any conclusive findings, the physician told her she was getting older and could not expect to feel as good as she did in her twenties. He then prescribed pain killers.

When the pain did not go away, the GP referred her to a gynecologist, who performed the same tests as well as a pelvic examination. Without any sign of organic damage, the second doctor also told her that her pain was age related. The woman expressed desperation, explaining that she could not sleep and had difficulty with work. So, she was referred to an orthopedist.

The third physician repeated the earlier testing and then referred her for a neurological examination. By this time, eight months had passed, and the woman was in so much pain that she could no longer perform her daily duties. The neurological tests did not provide any organic explanation for her pain. So, the neurologist advised her to consult with a psychiatrist. Instead, she went to Feldenkrais.

With a better appreciation for the link between the mind and body, Feldenkrais asked about her life experiences. She began her narrative with the fact that she had been in a concentration camp in Germany during WWII. While imprisoned she lost a child. She was liberated from the death camp as a 19-year-old child-adult. Because she had no way to earn money, she turned to prostitution. While living in France, she had a nervous breakdown (possibly precipitated by sexual violence).

Returning to her roots, she traveled from Europe to a kibbutz in Israel. There she started her life over, for a second time. Within a few years she remarried and had a baby boy. However, during the Israeli war both her husband and son were killed. Just prior to her current pelvic pain, she had reached the age of menopause, which meant that she could no longer give birth.

While explaining her experiences to Feldenkrais, the woman consciously concluded that she felt her emotional pain in the part of her body that had caused her the most suffering. This outcome fits with modern studies that have shown that the mind makes dual use of the neural correlates of physical and social pain. For example, Nathan DeWall and his colleagues (2015) have shown that regular doses of Tylenol can relieve hurt feelings from social rejection. In other words, there is a close relationship between psychic and physical pain.

Feldenkrais recognized this connection while also considering the symbolic significance of menopause (she could no longer make new life). As Feldenkrais (1981, 40–41) worded it, even though she had lived her life with extraordinary courage and vitality, she was now unfit to start her life again for a third time. Rather than judging her pain as bad or problematic, we can instead appreciate it as unconscious learning waiting to be utilized.

3.6 What to Observe

As demonstrated in Feldenkrais's case report, a comprehensive autobiographical narrative is indispensable to psychotherapeutics, especially when unconscious learnings and goals need to be considered. The autobiographical narrative enables us to observe behaviors that consequently illuminate emotional needs and thus choices made at unconscious levels.

Unfortunately, Feldenkrais did not describe how he helped this woman. We do know that he was willing to go to where her suffering was located—in the past. When helping someone who has been crippled by life's experiences, we do not ask them to come to us; rather, we bring the solution to where they are. In this case, it would mean going back to the woman's past and helping her recover her strength and vitality there.

Had it been my patient, I would have initiated unconscious process work by asking the question,

> What if you had not quit your work in the sex industry? What if you had never married or never discovered what it is to be a mother? Would your life have been better if you had chosen not to rebuild it?

I would then begin to talk about other clients and their progress (before she has a chance to reply), so that space is created for unconscious thought.

Given the evidence that conscious understanding of ourselves is derived mostly from other people's perceptions of us and in part from our own inferential guesswork, it is not surprising that we sometimes turn to others to help us make sense of ourselves. To better grasp this need, think of how sight works. Eyeballs collect information from objects out in front—nothing is seen on the interior. It seems consciousness is just as externally oriented.

Similarly, Freud argued that our true emotions were manifested in our behaviors, even if they were not represented in consciousness. If we take this idea one step further, it could be said that the true reasons for our actions are manifested in our behaviors—independent of conscious choice. Once this concept is understood, you can more skillfully observe yourself and others.

This reminds me of a man and a woman I once knew who decided to get together and read the Bible (the rationalization). He was married to someone else, as was she. Shortly into their Bible study, they decided to make margaritas. Eventually, they progressed from sipping margaritas on the balcony to the bedroom (the unconscious goal). Following their sexual encounter, neither of them could understand how their intention to study Christian principles led to the destruction of two marriages.

With events such as this, it seems that the best way to achieve introspection is to ignore our rationalizations for why we did something (or plan to do something) and instead look at the end produced by the behavior. A pragmatic question to ask one's self is, "If I saw someone else do this, what would I have to conclude was their motive?" In other words, meaningful self-knowledge is grounded in careful, accurate observations of our own behavior. It is like the dancer or yoga student. If she wishes to refine her movements, she must stand in front of a mirror and see what is happening or have a coach tell her what her body is doing.

What some consider Freud's greatest contribution to mental healing was the stand he took against scientific reductionism when he wrote in *Studies of Hysteria* (1895) that it is not enough to treat a patient's pathologies; rather, each individual has to be understood in terms of their life, their experience, and their story (Freud and Breuer, 1895). Conversely, what some consider Freud's greatest failing is his deterministic principles and clinical tendency to focus attention almost exclusively on an immutable past.

But the past has the same elastic qualities as the future. The human mind has a capacity for creativity and imagination that can literally reconfigure the past. Thus, it is just as reasonable to hope for a better past as it is to hope for a better future. As one client explained to me with relief,

> Before coming here, I didn't think you could change the past. That's why I didn't want to go to therapy. I thought it would be a waste of time. But you have made me realize, I can change the past by changing my interpretation of what happened! Now everything seems so different … It's hard to explain with words.

For this person, therapy not only consisted of reframing techniques but also an active engagement of unconscious reasoning capabilities. He had walked into a horrific scene, finding his friend's bloated body hanging from a rafter. The stench remained in his nostrils for days.

During therapy, this hard, seemingly immutable reality was broken down into pieces and subsequently rearranged as I asked a series of "what if" questions. These types of questions inspire imaginative creativity and generate new possibilities for the future. It also provides the opportunity to exercise choice in the face of tragedy. This evocation of imagination and creative reasoning is known in the research literature as *counterfactual thinking*. It is a creative potential that emerges as we reimagine the past or the future and have our choices witnessed by caring observers (this is a topic that will be taken up in greater detail in Chapter 7).

Chapter 3 Key Points

- Introspection is a guessing game. People naïvely reconstruct their explanations for behavior based on the available evidence.
- Unconscious intelligence is influenced by social values as it works to achieve discrete goals.
- Our most complex skill sets are based on a lifetime of implicit learning; thus, clients should be encouraged to trust what they know even without knowing how they know it.
- Conscious and unconscious functions can work separately or in unison.
- It is a mistake to label unconscious understandings as dysfunction when they do not conform to conscious logic.
- Self-knowledge must be grounded in careful, accurate observations of behavior(s), preferably with the help of outside observers—we come to know ourself through others.

References

Baars, Bernard J. 2005. "Global Workspace Theory of Consciousness: Toward a Cognitive Neuroscience of Human Experience." In *Progress in Brain Research*, 150, edited by Steven Laureys, 45–53. The Boundaries of Consciousness: Neurobiology and Neuropathology. Amsterdam: Elsevier. doi:10.1016/S0079-6123(05)50004-50009.

Bargh, John A., and Ezequiel Morsella. 2008. "The Unconscious Mind." *Perspectives on Psychological Science* 3 (1): 73–79. doi:10.1111/j.1745-6916.2008.00064.x.

Basch, M. F. 1976. "The Concept of Affect: A Re-Examination." *Journal of the American Psychoanalytic Association* 24 (4): 759–777. doi:10.1177/000306517602400401.

Baumeister, Roy F., and E. J. Masicampo. 2010. "Conscious Thought Is for Facilitating Social and Cultural Interactions: How Mental Simulations Serve the Animal–Culture Interface." *Psychological Review* 117 (3): 945–971. doi:10.1037/a0019393.

Bem, Daryl J. 1965. "An Experimental Analysis of Self-Persuasion." *Journal of Experimental Social Psychology* 1 (3): 199–218. doi:10.1016/0022-1031(65)90026-0.

Bowers, Kenneth S., Peter Farvolden, and Lambros Mermigis. 1995. "Intuitive Antecedents of Insight." In *The Creative Cognition Approach*, edited by Steven Smith, Thomas Ward, and Ronald Finke, 27–51. Boston, MA: MIT Press.

Damasio, Antonio R. 1999. *The Feeling of What Happens: Body and Emotion in the Making of Consciousness*. New York: Houghton Mifflin Harcourt.

Dehon, Erin, Nicole Weiss, Jonathan Jones, Whitney Faulconer, Elizabeth Hinton, and Sarah Sterling. 2017. "A Systematic Review of the Impact of Physician Implicit Racial Bias on Clinical Decision Making." *Academic Emergency Medicine* 24 (8): 895–904. doi:10.1111/acem.13214.

Dennett, Daniel C. 1982. "How to Study Human Consciousness Empirically or Nothing Comes to Mind." *Synthese* 53 (2): 159–180.

DeWall, Nathan C., David S. Chester, and Dylan S. White. 2015. "Can Acetaminophen Reduce the Pain of Decision-Making?" *Journal of Experimental Social Psychology* 56: 117–120. doi:10.1016/j.jesp.2014.09.006.

Erickson, Milton H. 1952. "Deep Hypnosis and Its Induction." In *Collected Works of Milton H. Erickson, Volume 1: The Nature of Therapeutic Hypnosis*, Vol. 1, edited by Ernest L. Rossi, Roxanna Erickson-Klein, and Kathryn Rossi, 1st edition, 229–260. Phoenix, AZ: Milton H. Erickson Foundation Press.

Erickson, Milton H. 1954. "A Clinical Note on Indirect Hypnotic Therapy." *Journal of Clinical and Experimental Hypnosis* 2 (3): 171–174. doi:10.1080/00207145408410051.

Erickson, Milton H. 1964. "The Burden of Responsibility in Effective Psychotherapy." *American Journal of Clinical Hypnosis* 6 (3): 269–271. doi:10.1080/00029157.1964.10402352.

Erickson, Milton H., Ernest L. Rossi, and Sheila I. Rossi. 1976. "Hypnotic Realities: The Induction of Clinical Hypnosis and Forms of Indirect Suggestion." In *Hypnotic Realities: The Induction of Clinical Hypnosis and Forms of Indirect Suggestion*. Vol. 10. Phoenix, AZ: Milton H. Erickson Foundation Press.

Feldenkrais, Moshé. 1981. *The Elusive Obvious: The Convergence of Movement, Neuroplasticity, and Health*. Cupertino, CA: Meta Publications.

Freud, Sigmund, and Joseph Breuer. (1895) 2004. *Studies in Hysteria*. New York: Penguin.

Glaser, Jack, and Mahzarin R. Banaji. 1999. "When Fair Is Foul and Foul Is Fair: Reverse Priming in Automatic Evaluation." *Journal of Personality and Social Psychology* 77 (4): 669–687. doi:10.1037/0022-3514.77.4.669.

Glaser, Jack, and John F. Kihlstrom. 2004. "Compensatory Automaticity: Unconscious Volition Is Not an Oxymoron." In *The New Unconscious*, edited by Ran R. Hassin, James S. Uleman, and John A. Bargh, 171–195. Oxford: Oxford University Press.

Greenberg, Leslie S. 2012. "Emotions, the Great Captains of Our Lives: Their Role in the Process of Change in Psychotherapy." *American Psychologist* 67 (8): 697–707. doi:10.1037/a0029858.

Haidt, Jonathan. 2001. "The Emotional Dog and Its Rational Tail: A Social Intuitionist Approach to Moral Judgment." *Psychological Review* 108 (4): 814–834. doi:10.1037/0033-295X.108.4.814.

Hall, Lars, Petter Johansson, and Thomas Strandberg. 2012. "Lifting the Veil of Morality: Choice Blindness and Attitude Reversals on a Self-Transforming Survey." *PLOS ONE* 7 (9): e45457. https://doi.org/10.1371/journal.pone.0045457.

Hume, David. 1800. *An Enquiry Concerning Human Understanding, An Enquiry Concerning the Principles of Morals, and The Natural History of Religion*. London: George Caw.

James, William. (1916) 1925. *Talks To Teachers On Psychology; And To Students On Some Of Life's Ideals.* New York: Henry Holt. Project Gutenberg. http://www.gutenberg.org/ebooks/16287.

Johansson, Petter, Lars Hall, Betty Tärning, Sverker Sikström, and Nick Chater. 2014. "Choice Blindness and Preference Change: You Will Like This Paper Better If You (Believe You) Chose to Read It!" *Journal of Behavioral Decision Making.* doi:10.1002/bdm.1807.

Jones, Ernest. 1908. "Rationalization in Every-Day Life." *The Journal of Abnormal Psychology* 3 (3): 161–169. doi:10.1037/h0070692.

Lewicki, Pawel. 1986. "Processing Information about Covariations That Cannot Be Articulated." *Journal of Experimental Psychology: Learning, Memory, and Cognition* 12 (1): 135–146. doi:10.1037/0278-7393.12.1.135.

Lewicki, Pawel, Maria Czyzewska, and Hunter Hoffman. 1987. "Unconscious Acquisition of Complex Procedural Knowledge." *Journal of Experimental Psychology: Learning, Memory, and Cognition* 13 (4): 523–530. doi:10.1037/0278-7393.13.4.523.

Lewicki, Pawel, Thomas Hill, and Maria Czyzewska. 1992. "Nonconscious Acquisition of Information." *American Psychologist* 47 (6): 796–801. doi:10.1037/0003-066X.47.6.796.

Myers, Frederic WilliamHenry. 1904. *Human Personality and Its Survival of Bodily Death.* Vol. 2. London: Forgotten Books.

Nisbett, Richard E., and Timothy D. Wilson. 1977. "Telling More than We Can Know: Verbal Reports on Mental Processes." *Psychological Review* 84 (3): 231–259. doi:10.1037/0033-295X.84.3.231.

North, Adrian C., David J. Hargreaves, and Jennifer McKendrick. 1999. "The Influence of In-Store Music on Wine Selections." *Journal of Applied Psychology* 84 (2): 271–276. doi:10.1037/0021-9010.84.2.271.

Oettingen, Gabriele, Heidi Grant, Pamela K. Smith, Mary Skinner, and Peter M. Gollwitzer. 2006. "Nonconscious Goal Pursuit: Acting in an Explanatory Vacuum." *Journal of Experimental Social Psychology* 42 (5): 668–675. doi:10.1016/j.jesp.2005.10.003.

Prince, Morton. 1912. *The Unconscious: The Fundamentals of Human Personality Normal and Abnormal.* New York: Macmillan.

Rubin, David C., Wanda T. Wallace, and Barbara C. Houston. 1993. "The Beginnings of Expertise for Ballads." *Cognitive Science* 17 (3): 435–462.

Stroop, J. R. 1935. "Studies of Interference in Serial Verbal Reactions." *Journal of Experimental Psychology* 18 (6): 643–662. doi:10.1037/h0054651.

Tanner, Robin J., Rosellina Ferraro, Tanya L. Chartrand, James R. Bettman, and Rick Van Baaren. 2008. "Of Chameleons and Consumption: The Impact of Mimicry on Choice and Preferences." *Journal of Consumer Research* 34 (6): 754–766. doi:10.1086/522322.

4 Motivation and Goal Setting

Adam Smith (1723–1790) used the analogy of an *invisible hand* to depict the influence of instinct on social behavior. As Smith (1776, 184) phrased it, "he intends only his own gain, and he is in this, as in many other cases, led by an invisible hand to promote an end which was no part of his intention." This metaphor works just as well when considering the effect of unconscious goal activation and the presence of habit. When clients come to therapy, they often describe their own actions as if they were guided by an invisible hand. A client of mine recently lamented,

> I do not know what is wrong with my brain. I tell myself to get to bed on time, but then I stay up till 2:00 a.m. watching TV. I tell myself to stick to my budget, but then I go online and purchase stuff I don't need.

As we have seen, situational cues can govern behavior without being consciously processed and without deliberate choice. Furthermore, situational cues that have been consistently and frequently associated with certain goals acquire the capacity to directly elicit unconscious goals and produce automatic behavior (implicit motivation).

The continuous activation of covert goals, learned through habit and triggered by situational cues, makes unconscious processes seem unintelligent and mechanistic. When clients find themselves automatically engaging in undesirable behavior, it can be demoralizing. This leads some clients to conclude, "How could I be so stupid?" In truth, the person may have pursued the hidden goal with great ingenuity and adaptive problem solving. The issue is not intelligence; rather, it is conflict created by the misalignment between conscious and unconscious problem-solving motives.

4.1 Unconscious Conflicts Do Not Register

The term *psychodynamic* generally refers to the idea that unconscious psychological forces impact behavior and development. Sigmund Freud's psychoanalysis was the original psychodynamic theory, but the psychodynamic approach to therapy is an umbrella term, which includes all theories that attend

DOI: 10.4324/9781003127208-4

to the interplay between conscious and unconscious processes, such as Carl Jung (Jung and Hinkle, 1921), Melanie Klein (1921), Wilhelm Reich (1925), Alfred Adler (1927), Anna Freud (1936), Karen Horney (1945), Erik Erikson (1950), Otto Kernberg (1975), and Milton Erickson (Erickson et al., 1976; Erickson and Rossi, 1979). Although this is only a partial list, it is still clear that most modern forms of psychotherapy have roots in psychodynamic psychology.

For Freud, the primary focus of treatment was intrapsychic conflicts (mostly sexual in nature), which he believed to be the chief cause of neuroticism. As Freud (1910) explains:

> In all those experiences [of cathartic treatment], it had happened that a wish had been aroused, which was in sharp opposition to the other desires of the individual, and was not capable of being reconciled with the ethical, aesthetic, and personal pretensions of the patient's personality. … This was, then, repressed from consciousness and forgotten.
>
> (7)

Freud's basic assumption was that motivational and affective processes operate simultaneously and in parallel at conscious and unconscious levels. In this regard, Freud was correct. This well-documented mental capability can result in individuals having conflicting feelings towards the same person or situation but without awareness.

In contrast, when a person feels ambivalent the conflicting goals or attitudes are fully known to conscious awareness. In Freudian theory, not only do psychodynamic conflicts remain unknown to conscious processes, but unconscious processes can also craft compromises outside of awareness in the form of defense mechanisms.

Expanding on Freud's understanding of the pivotal role relationships play in emotional health, Karen Horney (1945) argued that neurotic distress was an inevitable outgrowth of incompatibility between (a) conscious interpersonal strategies and (b) unconscious attitudes toward the self and others. According to Horney's theory, unconscious and conscious aspects of personality may work at cross purposes, producing motivational conflict and inconsistent behavior. As with Freud, Horney focuses on a psychodynamic conflict, meaning that the conflict is between explicit and implicit goals or attitudes.

Contemporary research into this type of intrapsychic conflict has supported Horney's theory. In one such study, it was found that automatic proximity seeking behavior (approach) can occur simultaneously with relational distancing (avoid) in the form of conscious devaluation of new partners. According to researchers Sommer and Bernieri (2015), the reason someone might devalue a person they are unconsciously drawn to might reflect efforts to minimize the potential for pain of future rejection. The same psychodynamic theory is often employed by parents seeking to console a confused child, "The reason Johnny calls you names and always steals your pencils is because he likes you." In other words, the child who has developed a strong attraction inexplicably begins to tease or physically harass the object of that desire.

Expanding our focus, we should recognize that conflicting attitudes are not limited to interactions with individuals. We can also be unknowingly conflicted over our attitudes towards self.

An important psychodynamic conflict for therapists to understand is the disparity that can occur between explicit and implicit self-esteem. The fact that researchers can reliably measure people's unconscious self-esteem is a fascinating topic unto itself. One such study by Bosson and colleagues (2003) found that people who scored relatively high on an explicit measure of self-esteem, but relatively low on an implicit measure, exhibited the most self-aggrandizement across different indices. This fits with other studies that found similarities between narcissistic personality and those with conscious positive self-attitudes combined with unconscious negative self-attitudes. Other characteristics, such as hypersensitivity to criticism, tendency to use blame, and low emotional self-awareness can all be predicted after identifying this set of psychodynamics (Jordan et al., 2003; Shedler et al., 1993).

People can also be conflicted over their attitudes towards a group of individuals. For example, numerous studies have shown that people who consider themselves non-racist sometimes have two or more conflicting sets of attitudes that influence their behavior. At a conscious level, they are most likely to experience socially endorsed attitudes (anti-prejudiced); but at an unconscious level, negative attitudes towards skin color do exist. Furthermore, these conscious and unconscious racial attitudes can operate completely independent of each other (Gaertner et al., 1993).

More specifically, Banaji and Hardin (1996) found that a measure of unconscious negative attitudes will predict how likely it is that a person who considers herself non-racist would be rated as friendly by an African-American interviewer (automatic behavior). Yet these unconscious associations will not predict conscious attitudes when the individual is asked questions about racial inequality in the United States (effortful conscious intention). Those attitudes are best predicted using a measure of explicit attitudes on race. Though not Freudian, this is a psychodynamic conflict.

What therapists can learn from these studies is that when people are focusing on their conscious attitudes, their behavior will reflect these explicit attitudes; however, they are not carried over to spontaneous interactions. For example, when a husband is trying to explain to his therapist that he does not have any negative attitudes towards women (though he has a history of treating women scornfully), his behavior will be influenced by his explicit attitudes. While discussing the topic, he uses charitable language and respectful behavior towards his partner and/or female therapist. However, during the stress and distractions of everyday life, unconscious affective associations and negative attitudes guide his actions, causing him to be disapproving and subtly antagonistic towards his wife. Implicit sexism can result in him using negative stereotypes, such as "Just like a woman to be so manipulative!" These little slices of behavior act as a window, exposing implicit attitudes and unconscious goals.

The temptation is to assume this person is lying to his therapist or being resistant to therapy. But we should not be so judgmental. It is equally possible that our client is only identifying with those attitudes that reside within conscious awareness—literally, the only behavior he is paying attention to.

This brings us to the Freudian concept of resistance, which commonly occurs when therapists try to inform clients that they are suffering from psychodynamic conflicts. According to Freud, clients resist these interpretations of their behavior because they are defensively seeking to prevent repressed information from emerging into consciousness. Another possibility is that the high inference interpretations are resisted because they are inaccurate. Yet another possibility is that a mental conflict may exist, but the client rejected the idea simply because these conflicts do not register in conscious awareness.

A point that can hardly be overstated is that psychodynamic conflicts are not known to the individual. We see this in studies on implicit racism. One such study conducted by Greenwald and Schuh (1994) examined reference citation behavior among social scientists and researchers who study prejudice. In other words, they looked for signs of implicit racism in a group of people consciously dedicated to addressing the problem of racism. But when looking at the names of the authors cited in their papers, the study found that authors were approximately 40% more likely to cite colleagues from their own ethnic category. This is remarkable when we consider that, of all people, researchers studying prejudice should be especially aware of the influence of unconscious attitudes and highly motivated to pursue fair and equal treatment.

Had these subjects been interviewed, it is highly likely that the behavior would have been rationalized based on ethnic involvement in a given specialty area (I couldn't find any Jews who published on this topic) or personal acquaintance (I am friends with these researchers). However, these variables were statistically controlled, and nonetheless the results revealed an implicit bias against members of a religious outgroup.

Lastly, if two conscious goals can be in conflict (ambivalence), then can multiple unconscious goals also be in conflict (implicit ambivalence)? The answer seems to be yes. In a recent test of non-conscious goal pursuit, Tali Kleiman and Ran Hassin (2011) demonstrated that two goals can in fact be in active conflict outside of conscious awareness. Under these conditions the subjects did not experience any explicit changes in felt conflict. The individuals were presumably healthy and unimpeded by defense mechanisms.

The clinical implications for implicit ambivalence are currently unknown. My best guess is that when this type of conflict occurs, it impedes spontaneity in the same way that conscious ambivalence inhibits intentional action (forcing us to stop and deliberate before acting). What is abundantly clear is that a wide variety of psychodynamic conflicts exist beyond the reach of introspection.

4.2 Motivation is an Amalgamation of Conscious and Unconscious Goals

Next we turn to research on motivation, which answers the question of why people act, in which direction, and with how much intensity. The hedonic principle (people approach pleasure and avoid pain) has remained the foundational motivational principle throughout the history of psychology. This basic dichotomy (that can be traced back to Plato) has been explored and elaborated in terms of intrinsic/extrinsic motivation (we work harder and longer for goals aimed at internal rewards), loss aversion motivation (we work harder to prevent loss than to pursue gain), promotion focus versus a prevention focus (we are happier and more effective when pursuing positive outcomes rather than seeking to prevent negative outcomes), and temporal motivational theory (TMT) (we are more likely to pursue goals or tasks that are pleasurable and that we are likely to attain, while we are more likely to put off or procrastinate difficult tasks with unenjoyable qualities).

Many of the factors listed above will simultaneously influence behavior, often without conscious awareness and in some instances in conflict with conscious logic. For example, imagine what would happen when young heterosexual males are primed with romantic goals (unconsciously) and then given a choice to take a course given by a male or female instructor. What Bar-Anan and colleagues (2010) found was that young men primed with romantic goals both rated their liking for the female-taught topic significantly higher and endorsed more highly the idea that they were the kind of person who was interested in her topic (than those with no sexual goal prime). When asked to explain these choices, everyone produced a rationalized response, one that fit with their conscious goals and objectives (a classic psychodynamic conflict: motivated by sex but justified by higher social values).

In most clinical cases, rather than asking whether a person is experiencing psychodynamic conflicts, the more pertinent clinical questions are about how many motivational forces might be impacting a single point of choice, and how unrecognized conflict can be reduced. For example, what if a woman decided to marry one man because he was rich and handsome, but she had an unconscious affection for a different man? We can get some interesting ideas by looking at a brief case report from Milton Erickson (Erickson and Rosen, 1982).

While conducting a lecture on hypnosis at Michigan State University in 1959, Erickson had a student volunteer a problem. She said, "I have some hideous secret, and I don't want to know it … but I ought to know it. … Can you do anything about it?" Erickson answered that he could. All she needed to do was take a pencil in her hand and, while looking at him, let her hand write this troublesome secret automatically. Erickson sat at the far end of the table with everyone else so that only she knew (unconsciously) what was written. Without looking down, she wrote a question to herself: "Will I marry Harold?"

We can assume that she was motivated to discover her secret because she did write it down. But she was just as motivated to hide the secret, so without conscious awareness she folded the piece of paper several times and slipped it into her purse. Next, Erickson suggested she enter a trance state and automatically write, "It's a beautiful day in June." It was April.

After she was awakened, Erickson showed her the automatic handwriting, but she insisted she had not written it because it wasn't her handwriting. Erickson agreed that it did not look like her handwriting.

Before continuing with the case narrative, let us consider the motivational dimensions of Erickson's prime. The phrase, "It's a beautiful day in June" is entirely open ended. If her unconscious identifies a goal, it will be one that she constructed to meet her needs (intrinsic motivation). What we know from recent research is that compelling goals can be activated outside of conscious awareness, and goal-directed behaviors can be triggered and deployed also without awareness (Hassin et al., 2004). In the case of this woman, such a goal would cause her to work, without her conscious knowledge, to achieve the desired outcome in June. Furthermore, she would likely become increasingly motivated as the June deadline approaches. According to TMT theory, the perceived usefulness and benefit of an activity increases exponentially as the deadline for completion nears.

Erickson reports that the girl called him from Indiana the following September. She said,

> A funny thing happened today, and I think you're connected with it—so I'll tell you what it is. I emptied my handbag today. I found a wad of paper in it. I opened it, and on one side was written in a strange handwriting, "Will I marry Harold?" It wasn't my handwriting. I don't know how that paper got into my handbag. And I have a feeling you're connected with it. ... Do you have any explanation of that piece of paper?

Erickson replied, "I lectured at the university in April; that's true. Now, were you by chance engaged to get married to anybody then?" She replied, "Oh yes, I was engaged to Bill." Erickson asked her if she had felt any doubts about marrying Bill. She said that she had no doubts until June, when she suddenly broke off the engagement. Erickson then asked, "What has happened since then?" She answered, "In July, I married a man named Harold."

Curious, Erickson asked, "How long had you known Harold?" She explained that she had only caught a glimpse of Harold earlier in the Spring semester. It was not until July that she began speaking with Harold.

Erickson interpreted these events, telling the woman that her unconscious mind had already recognized that she had doubts about her engagement to Bill and that she was interested in Harold (Erickson and Rossi, 1982). He surmised that the reason she folded up the message and hid it in her purse was because, consciously, she could not stand facing that fact in April.

It seems that her unconscious intelligence concluded that she was preparing to marry the wrong person. This conflict did not register in conscious awareness, however, until June. Still, she sought out hypnosis, and during a moment of unconscious process work she wrote herself a question that served as her own prime for future conscious consideration (unconscious planning). As for her only catching a glimpse of Harold, researchers have found that people are often surprisingly accurate when making judgments of others based on mere glimpses. Very brief samples, or "thin slices," produce a surprising amount of unconscious knowledge that can lead to accurate emotional forecasting (Ambady et al., 2000).

4.3 Utilizing Cognitive Dissonance

In social psychology, cognitive dissonance is said to occur when a person has beliefs, ideas, or values that contradict his or her observed behaviors. The general finding in this body of research is that there are processes of unconscious self-regulation that will automatically seek to reduce intrapsychic conflict by changing attitudes or beliefs to align with observed behaviors. Interestingly, individuals do not know that they are making these adjustments; therefore, if there is distress or discomfort caused by internal conflict, it may not be known to conscious awareness. The way to utilize this phenomenon (cognitive dissonance) in psychotherapy is to help guide conscious awareness to behaviors that are useful for establishing new implicit attitudes, values, and goals.

If I listen to a client describe a story of a close friend whose marriage is in serious trouble (a probable projection), and then I ask, "What does your friend need to do immediately to get his marriage back on track?" The question will draw attention to the possibility of a catastrophic outcome. I am not forcing an analytic interpretation on his conscious awareness because his unconscious is already attending to the issue. My statement is meant to make the situation feel urgent, an effort to activate unconscious processes aimed at increased security. This occurs because the wording of the question activates mental representations associated with obligations and the threat of loss. Outside of conscious awareness, a counter question is cued, "How might this apply to me?"

This leads to the type of motivation known as prevention-focus (security priority), which is known to evoke greater commitment, certainty, and careful, vigilant analysis. In its most extreme form, it creates a nagging sense of anxiety or self-consciousness (Molden and Lee, 2008).

This is the type of motivation I would choose for a domestic violence situation when seeking to help the aggressor. Because increased anxiety and self-consciousness (security seeking) is incompatible with anger (high risk tolerance), it has practical value in these circumstances. As one client stated to me, "I'm not violent anymore, which is good, but I am constantly thinking about my actions, wondering if I might have done something to upset her." In other words, his implicit attitudes had come into line with his conscious goal of no longer using violence in the relationship.

While working with one such individual, I primed him for a lengthy process of resolving shame issues while increasing his implicit self-esteem by saying,

> Given the amount of harm that you have inflicted on her, you will be lucky if you are able to save the marriage. Most men cannot. You certainly will *not* be able to save the marriage by being an average good husband. Given what has happened, your actions will need to prove, over a long period of time, that you are an above average husband.

If he consistently acts in a way that she perceives as good, then the associated label (above average husband) will help his unconscious self-esteem increase. Even more importantly, these behaviors are likely to alter implicit attitudes toward his wife. According to cognitive dissonance theory, if he is treating her exceptionally well, then it must mean she has extraordinary value (automatic alignment). This is what his wife had been doing all along (treating him like a king), and why she so deeply valued him, up until reaching her breaking point.

It is interesting to note that research on racism has shown that people can dramatically reduce their implicit bias simply by relabeling their intended actions toward out groups (as caring or protective actions). In other words, how people label their intended actions may shape the outcomes of their social interactions by dramatically altering their attitudes and emotions towards others (Melnikoff et al., 2020). This is a special instance of cognitive dissonance such that implicit self-regulatory processes are seeking to align attitudes with imagined actions. Thus, if a person labels his behavior as caring, then he is more likely to construct mental representations of caring behavior, which will then cause implicit attitudes to automatically shift in that direction.

If we apply this utilization of cognitive dissonance to implicit self-esteem, then having a person label his actions as attempts to express esteem-worthy values should produce a similar effect. If I help a client construct a lengthy and detailed account of how he is endeavoring to treat his wife in a loving way, that process is likely to shift some of his implicit values not only towards valuing her but himself as well.

This approach is very different from offering free-floating general praise, such as the statement, "You are a good person." A person who is narcissistic will devour that message and be no better for it. Instead, when you carefully examine discrete actions and expose them to the possibility of negative labeling, it puts the client in a vulnerable position (showing you could confirm his worst fears—that he is deeply flawed). When the client realizes that he is not in control of your attention (because you ignore his use of blame, denial, and/or projection), it is as if you have stripped away the veneer of pseudo self-confidence, and a fragile self is exposed.

If the individual can tolerate this vulnerable state, and you treat him with care, then a new personality begins to emerge. My experience is that this surgical dissection of his actions has a therapeutic influence if you protect the fragile parts and appeal to his nobler aspirations. The individual starts to act less narcissistically as his implicit self-esteem starts to elevate and his explicit self-esteem lowers to a more functional level. This occurs when I help him become more fluent in confessing mistakes and learning from them (lowering explicit self-esteem) while applying positive labels to his intended behavior (raising implicit self-esteem), thus the psychodynamic conflict is reduced.

This approach to implicit self-esteem work can also be described as a benevolent interpretation: "I see your actions, I am willing to describe them in concrete detail, and I will assign a charitable label so that this can become your new implicit goal." It is reminiscent of the transformation we see in Victor Hugo's *Les Misérables* (1862) when Bishop Myriel says to Jean Valjean (after his thieving actions are exposed), "never forget that you have promised to use this money in becoming an honest man" (ch. 12).

In therapy, I may say to a domestic violence client,

> You did yell at your wife this past week. Your face probably looked angrier and more hostile than you would have wished. The fact that you feel ashamed to tell me about this means you are developing a stronger conscience (new implicit goal = develop a stronger conscience).

In contrast, if I were working with a kind husband with neurotic struggles, I might ask, "If your wife was to come into my office five years from now, what would you like her to say about you … the things that set you apart from any other husband?" Similarly, I recently asked a client to close his eyes and then *see* the answer to this question: "If your wife outlived you, and she was at the funeral reading your eulogy to a room full of people, what would you want to appear in that eulogy?" Both questions focus the client on his actions and prime groundbreaking work. There are now thirty years of accumulated studies showing that different types of goals activate different motivational structures. This last imaginative exercise is aimed at a distant future with abstract goals. This contrasts with the domestic violence example in which my question was aimed at an immediate future with urgent concrete goals—save the marriage. Furthermore, there is an emphasis on individuation and an idealized self, in contrast to the earlier example that focused on social obligations.

This different line of questioning leads to the type of motivation known as promotion-focus (achievement priority), which has been shown in research to evoke greater flexibility, open-mindedness, and speedy, eager progress. In its most extreme form, promotion-focus creates a sense of excitement with a greater tolerance for risks and persistence in the face of obstacles (Molden and Lee, 2008). This is the type of unconscious motivation I would choose for any non-crisis situation.

It is important to note that if we wish to involve unconscious process work, then we do not wait for emotionally provocative questions to be answered. If time is provided for conscious deliberation, then conscious process work starts to dominate. This reminds me of a conversation with Milton Erickson's daughter, Roxanna Erickson, who told me that her father would often change the topic of conversation immediately after hypnosis because he believed that for unconscious processing to occur, conscious analysis should not be allowed to hijack the process. Erickson Rossi, and Rossi (1976) argued against building "associative bridges" when engaging unconscious processes. Roxanna compared this prohibition to shaking Jell-O before it has had time to set. With any sensory input at any level of complexity, the mind seeks completion. This was demonstrated repeatedly in the early studies on Gestalt psychology. Questions will be answered—if not at conscious levels, then at unconscious levels.

4.4 Goals are Like Instincts, They Get Triggered

Because Freud (1900) equated unconscious motives with instinctual drives, he assumed that they are always active. In contrast, researchers such as Bargh (1990) and Wilson (2004) have argued for the importance of disentangling cognitive motives from primitive motives, which can both operate on conscious or unconscious levels. When this distinction is made, researchers have found that unconscious motives (goal-oriented, emotion-driven processes) will not influence behavior unless something has activated them. Having studied a great deal of ethnology, I would make the additional point that instincts must also be triggered before influencing behavior.

If we think of both instinctual behavior and goal-oriented behavior as action potentials waiting to be triggered, then it provides an interesting explanation for some of the advantages of clinical hypnosis over traditional process work. One of the great benefits of hypnotic suggestion might be its ability to activate unconscious goals and motivation in a way that synchronizes with conscious needs and goals. If we compare psychodynamic conflicts to a room full of noisy people (there can be more than one conflict), then the value of a choir director has obvious implications for psychotherapy. From this perspective, unconscious process work is seen as a strategic effort to create harmony between conscious and unconscious motives.

Thus, one of the crucial tasks in therapy is to activate a meaningful goal so that unconscious processes can organize problem-solving activity around it. It is in this endeavor that the practices of psychotherapy and hypnotherapy converge. Looking back to Bargh's (1990) groundbreaking work, there are now thirty years of accumulated studies showing that goals can be activated without conscious awareness, even in non-hypnotic contexts, and they are then pursued unconsciously with tenacity and persistence. Similar to what we see in Erickson's work, researchers have found that unconscious goal pursuit (which is triggered by simply having a word, such as cooperation, appear several times in written material) can enhance sensitivity to relevant aspects of the environment, and it can enhance cognitive and behavioral flexibility (Ferguson et al., 2008).

When dealing with a disharmonious mind, there is an advantage to be found in having an overarching goal that operates outside of conscious awareness. Returning to our example from Erickson, we can ask, "Would it not have been just as easy for him to ask the woman if she was about to make any big decisions?" And, when she says she is engaged, then ask her, "Are you certain this is the right person for you? Have you really stopped to think about all your options?"

The question is not entirely hypothetical. I had a friend who was in a similar situation. Her best friend became engaged to someone she had hardly started dating. The best friend felt rushed because all of her younger sisters had already married. A caring discussion about the certainty of her choice did not go well; the bride-to-be never spoke to my friend again. Twelve months later I saw that the marriage had already ended in divorce. The concerns had been warranted, but the friendship was never restored.

In my practice, I frequently receive new clients who were in therapy with someone else but quit just as soon as they were presented with a goal that they consciously did not wish to consider. By the time a client gets to me, she might confess, "I think that therapist could be right. But I didn't want to see her again after she said that." If I wish to help the client, then I had better support her unconscious goals and motivations, but outside of conscious awareness (i.e., she would not have sought out a second therapist if there was not a conflict between her conscious and unconscious motivations).

Accordingly, laboratory tests have shown that unconscious goals may lead people to work harder than they would for a conscious goal (less resistance to being told what to do). For example, Bargh and colleagues (2001) demonstrated that an unconsciously activated achievement goal (subliminal priming) caused experiment participants to work longer and harder on assigned word puzzles. In fact, the majority of the goal-primed participants continued working on the puzzles even after they were supposed to stop, illustrating a concern with achieving the highest possible score. This is the reaction we would expect when people feel intrinsically motivated—a clear advantage of unconscious goal activation.

Another important advantage is the ubiquitous nature of unconscious motivation. As shown by Bargh and colleagues (2001), the goal concept, once activated without the participant's awareness, operates over extended time periods to guide thought or behavior towards the goal. Remarkably, these processes do not require conscious intent or monitoring. Even more interestingly, it has been found that unconscious motives increase in strength until acted on. They produce persistence at task performance in the face of obstacles, and they favor resumption of disrupted tasks, even in the presence of more attractive alternatives.

This contrasts with conscious, explicit motives that influence behavior only when conscious attention is focused on them. Shortly after doing so, the spotlight of conscious attention fades (as energy is depleted) or shifts to the first distraction. Thus, effortful goal pursuit is notoriously short-lived.

When considering how difficult it might be to activate unconscious goals in the clinical setting, it is worth noting that researchers were able to influence people's behavior in social situations simply by having them read words that were synonymous with the goal (no altered states of consciousness needed).

For example, Bargh and others (2001) showed that a goal to be considerate can be unconsciously activated by simply reading related words, such as "cooperate," which caused participants playing the role of a fishing company to voluntarily put more fish back into a lake to replenish the fish population (thereby reducing their own profits) compared to participants in a control condition.

While these results sometimes fail to replicate (Cesario, 2014), it is worth noting that in the therapy setting exposure is dramatically increased (you can continue the persistent use of primes for dozens of visits). While highly suggestible clients respond immediately to primes, predictions, and suggestions, others require longer exposure and more time to establish the therapeutic alliance.

Therapists who decorate their offices with words such as "hope" and "resiliency" can expect to achieve similar effects—especially when problems are disclosed for which these goals have great relevance. While working in front of bookshelves filled with self-help literature, I sometimes see a client glance in the direction of the vertical book titles. If asked "What just caught your eye?", the client might reply, "I keep looking at that book, the one titled *I'm OK—You're OK*."

Sometimes, when I see that the client is having a meaningful reaction to something, I will direct conscious attention to the experience (conscious process work). For example, asking what she thinks about a book title, an image on the wall, or a gap sentence. I do this so that I can better understand what ideas are emotionally important to the client. Also, conscious awareness might help integrate unconscious goals with conscious motivation. However, there are instances in which conscious attention to an unconscious process can impede progress.

Specifically, we should not attempt to elicit conscious goal-oriented activity when emotionality is high and unconscious motivation is available. According to controlled experimentation, when conscious motives are activated, they tend to override unconscious motives and guide behavior using less complex and less well-established skill sets.

In therapy, we need to fully encourage spontaneous behavior and gut-level responses whenever possible. This is one of the great benefits of the hypnosis paradigm. Equipped with the expectation that benefits will occur automatically, the hypnotherapy client does not seek to engage conscious intention. It is the difference between leaning into spontaneity and automatic behaviors (just let it happen) versus effortful intention (make it happen).

As shown by McClelland and colleagues (1989), when conscious goals are not active, unconscious goals govern behavior. Because unconscious representations have the greatest capacity for sustained operations across far larger periods of time, their governing force is superior. But that does not mean that conscious motives cannot interrupt and temporarily govern the process. This power-sharing arrangement can be informed by science. As we will see in Chapter 9, there are certain instances when conscious analysis is more effective than unconscious analysis. I have found that clients appreciate being told when to deliberate and when to just go with what they intuitively know.

4.5 Planning Automatic Behavior

Because planning reduces conflict, it is something we should consider when discussing psychodynamic conflicts. When seeking to better understand the pros and cons of conscious deliberation, it is important to recognize differences between novel goals versus habitual pursuits. Novel goals require conscious deliberation, while familiar goals become linked to automatic, experience-based behavior. For novel goals we must stop to consider options, perhaps learn new skills, and develop a plan for how to achieve the desired end. But for those goals that are pursued routinely (such as tasks performed at work) conscious attention is eliminated.

These are not new ideas. William James saw the great value of automatic behavior and described habit as playing a pivotal role in the pursuit of a healthy life. As James (1916) states, "All our life, so far as it has definite form, is but a mass of habits—practical, emotional, intellectual—systematically organized for our weal or woe, and bearing us irresistibly toward our destiny, whatever the latter may be" (64).

Destiny is not always the thing an individual may have consciously chosen. As an example of people's destinies being governed by habit, James (1914, 50) observes, "Men grown old in prison have asked to be readmitted after being once set free." As explained by Aarts and Dijksterhuis (2000), habits can be seen as hieratical mental representations in which activation of a goal leads to activation of many other behaviors lower in the hierarchy. The result is a bundled set of skilled behaviors that are linked to a particular goal or to a particular dimension of our personal identity.

The practical application of this hierarchy for psychotherapy was described by Erickson (1959) in a method he called *transference of learning*. This technique acts as a bridge so that unconscious learning and motivations that have become associated with one context can be moved over to a new context.

As an example, I had a man come to me and request help with his marriage. The problem was he felt horribly disempowered and was unable to assert himself while dealing with his controlling wife. As a result, he was resentful, withdrawn, and only emotionally at peace when he travelled for work.

I asked him to describe his profession. His voice suddenly became solemn as he said, "I'm a fixer." Sounding a little bit like a mafia hitman, he continued, "When a corporation is not working right, the board will hire me to come in and fix things." Curious, I asked, "What if the CEO does not want to implement the new changes?"

I knew we were talking about the CEOs of large companies headquartered in New York, so these would be exceedingly dominant individuals. He replied with a cool glance and an allusive nod, "They never tell me no. Their jobs depend on it." Having activated a relevant skill set, I asked him, "If you were to go home as the fixer, and have a talk with your wife, what would you say?" Without hesitation, he replied,

> I would say that she is unhappy, and I am unhappy. I would tell her that I do not want a divorce, so I will lease an apartment down the street. I will come to the house on the weekends to help with the pool and other chores.

In order for me to appreciate the logic behind his fix, he went on to explain,

> She is a good mother. I want her to live comfortably in the home with our 11-year-old son. She has never worked and would not know how to enter the job market. I will continue to pay all the bills. I just cannot continue living in the same house as her.

The transformation in personality was stunning. No hypnosis was used. He was simply primed to activate the mental representations linked to being "a fixer." The cognitive skills that suddenly appeared were complex and nuanced. Any effort to teach all of this (experiential knowledge and emotional disposition) to his conscious awareness would have taken months, if not longer.

Although it seems that people should consciously know how much they know—and be ready to use it—most often, this is not the case. This brings us back to Bargh's proposition that unconscious goals will not influence behavior unless something has activated them.

Unfortunately, the transference of learning (linking) is not always an option. When an established skill set is not readily available, the next best thing to do is to develop a step-by-step plan that is rehearsed in roleplay or guided imagery exercises. According to researchers, planning is like habit formation in that it also creates hieratical mental representations in which specific behaviors are linked for the purpose of achieving an overarching goal. This strategy has been studied experimentally in terms of *prepared reflexes*. In this approach new automatic behaviors are set up by strategically using "if then" statements that are connected to external stimuli.

For example, while working with a client who has used violence in the marriage, I can say, "If next week your wife becomes angry at you and you respond with humility, then she will get to see that you have *become stronger* on the inside." To trigger unconscious goal-pursuit, the words chosen need to have special emotional significance to the client. In order to overcome problematic habits (such as anger), the new associations formed through planning for a novel goal (something incompatible with anger) must be stronger than the habitual associations. In this example, the words "become stronger" will be embraced automatically by someone who greatly values strength.

When setting up prepared reflexes it is also important to establish a trigger for goal implementation. According to research, a prepared reflex will automatically guide behavior if it is held in unconscious working memory.

This is achieved by using an upcoming event as a point of reference—something that creates anticipation.

In my example, if the man has complained that his wife is starting to show her anger (now that she is less frightened of him), then that is a point of reference I can use to keep the new unconscious goal active. In this case, the new behavior of responding with humility is now dependent on an external cue—his wife becoming angry. If the novel goal is motivationally appealing, then the goal-oriented behavior will activate at the right moment without effortful conscious thought (Melnikoff et al., 2020).

If I wish to establish the new goal even more powerfully in unconscious working memory, then I can add an element of suspense. For example, I might say, "You never know when someone will get angry with you. It could happen tomorrow or three months from now. But when it does happen, it will be a pop quiz, and you will either pass or fail."

As another example, I can say to an overly inhibited client,

> Now that you have practiced asserting your needs in here with me, and competently so, it will be much easier to do the same at work. So, the next time your boss wants to talk [stimulus trigger], you will be able to look him in the eyes and speak confidently [goal response].

Here I have combined the use of prediction with a prepared reflex. My statement sounds like a post-hypnotic suggestion because the dynamics are the same (this concept will be revisited in Chapter 6).

Chapter 4 Key Points

- Because psychodynamic conflicts cannot be sensed by conscious awareness, their influence cannot be resolved by conscious reason or analytic interpretations.
- Many different forms of motivation can simultaneously influence behavior, often without conscious awareness and in some instances in conflict with conscious logic.
- Some questions are best left unanswered. This promotes unconscious process work.
- Priming or suggestion helps activate unconscious goals that fit with conscious objectives.
- Planning to use existing skill sets in new contexts, under specific conditions, helps establish spontaneous coping.

References

Aarts, Henk, and Ap Dijksterhuis. 2000. "Habits as Knowledge Structures: Automaticity in Goal-Directed Behavior." *Journal of Personality and Social Psychology* 78 (1): 53–63. doi:10.1037/0022-3514.78.1.53.

Adler, Alfred. 1927. *Understanding Human Nature*. New York: Garden City Publishing.

Ambady, Nalini, Frank J. Bernieri, and Jennifer A. Richeson. 2000. "Toward a Histology of Social Behavior: Judgmental Accuracy from Thin Slices of the Behavioral Stream." In *Advances in Experimental Social Psychology*, Vol. 32, edited by Mark P. Zanna, 201–271. San Diego, CA: Academic Press. doi:10.1016/S0065-2601(00)80006–80004.

Banaji, Mahzarin R., and Curtis D. Hardin. 1996. "Automatic Stereotyping." *Psychological Science* 7 (3): 136–141. doi:10.1111/j.1467-9280.1996.tb00346.x.

Bar-Anan, Yoav, Timothy D. Wilson, and Ran R. Hassin. 2010. "Inaccurate Self-Knowledge Formation as a Result of Automatic Behavior." *Journal of Experimental Social Psychology* 46 (6): 884–894. doi:10.1016/j.jesp.2010.07.007.

Bargh, John A. 1990. "Goal and Intent: Goal-Directed Thought and Behavior Are Often Unintentional." *Psychological Inquiry* 1 (3): 248–251. doi:10.1207/s15327965pli0103_14.

Bargh, John A., Peter M. Gollwitzer, Annette Lee-Chai, Kimberly Barndollar, and Roman Trötschel. 2001. "The Automated Will: Nonconscious Activation and Pursuit of Behavioral Goals." *Journal of Personality and Social Psychology* 81 (6): 1014–1027. doi:10.1037/0022-3514.81.6.1014.

Bosson, Jennifer K., Ryan P. Brown, Virgil Zeigler-Hill, and William B. Swann. 2003. "Self-Enhancement Tendencies Among People With High Explicit Self-Esteem: The Moderating Role of Implicit Self-Esteem." *Self and Identity* 2 (3): 169–187. doi:10.1080/15298860309029.

Cesario, Joseph. 2014. "Priming, Replication, and the Hardest Science." *Perspectives on Psychological Science* 9 (1): 40–48. doi:10.1177/1745691613513470.

Erickson, Milton H. 1959. "The Basis of Hypnosis: Panel Discussion on Hypnosis." In *Collected Works of Milton H. Erickson, Volume 8: General and Historical Surveys of Hypnosis*, edited by Ernest L. Rossi, Roxanna Erickson-Klein, and Kathryn Rossi, 35–42. Phoenix, AZ: Milton H. Erickson Foundation Press.

Erickson, Milton H., and Sidney Rosen. 1982. *My Voice Will Go with You: The Teaching Tales of Milton H. Erickson, MD*. New York: W. W. Norton & Company.

Erickson, Milton H., and Ernest L. Rossi. 1979. *Hypnotherapy: An Exploratory Casebook*. Har/Cas edition. New York: Irvington Pub.

Erickson, Milton H., Ernest L. Rossi, and Sheila I. Rossi. 1976. *Hypnotic Realities: The Induction of Clinical Hypnosis and Forms of Indirect Suggestion*, Vol. 10. Phoenix, AZ: Milton H. Erickson Foundation Press.

Erikson, Erik H. 1950. *Childhood and Society*. New York: W. W. Norton & Company.

Ferguson, Melissa J., Ran Hassin, and John A.Bargh. 2008. "Implicit Motivation: Past, Present, and Future." In *Handbook of Motivation Science*, edited by J. Shah and W. Gardner, 150–166. New York: The Guilford Press.

Freud, Anna. (1936) 1950. *The Ego and the Mechanisms of Defense*. Revised Edition, Tenth Printing edition. New York: International Universities Press.

Freud, Sigmund. (1900) 1966. "The Interpretation Of Dreams." In *The Basic Writings of Sigmund Freud*, translated and edited by A. A. Brill, 181–468. New York: Random House.

Freud, Sigmund. (1910) 1955. The Origin and Development of Psychoanalysis. In *An Outline of Psychoanalysis*, edited by J. S. Van Teslaar, 21–70. New York: Modern Library. doi:10.1037/11350-001.

Gaertner, Samuel L., John F. Dovidio, Phyllis A. Anastasio, Betty A. Bachman, and Mary C. Rust. 1993. "The Common Ingroup Identity Model: Recategorization and the Reduction of Intergroup Bias." *European Review of Social Psychology* 4 (1): 1–26. doi:10.1080/14792779343000004.

Greenwald, Anthony, and Eric S. Schuh. 1994. "An Ethnic Bias in Scientific Citations." *European Journal of Social Psychology* 24: 623–639.

Hassin, Ran R., James S. Uleman, and John A. Bargh, eds. 2004. *The New Unconscious*. Oxford: Oxford University Press.

Horney, Karen. (1945) 1993. *Our Inner Conflicts: A Constructive Theory of Neurosis*. New York: Norton.

Hugo, Victor. (1862) 1887. *Les Misérables*. Translated by Isabel F. Hapgood. New York: Thomas Y. Crowell. Project Gutenberg. http://www.gutenberg.org/files/135/135-h/135-h.htm.

James, William. 1914. *Habit*. New York: Henry Holt.

James, William. (1916) 1925. *Talks To Teachers On Psychology; And To Students On Some Of Life's Ideals*. New York: Henry Holt. Project Gutenberg. http://www.gutenberg.org/ebooks/16287.

Jordan, Christian H., Steven J. Spencer, Mark P. Zanna, Etsuko Hoshino-Browne, and Joshua Correll. 2003. "Secure and Defensive High Self-Esteem." *Journal of Personality and Social Psychology* 85 (5): 969–978. doi:10.1037/0022-3514.85.5.969.

Jung, Carl Gustav, and Beatrice M. Hinkle. 1921. *Psychology of the Unconscious: A Study of the Transformations and Symbolisms of the Libido ; a Contribution to the History of the Evolution of Thought*. New York: Moffat, Yard & Company.

Kernberg, Otto F. 1975. *Borderline Conditions and Pathological Narcissism*. Reissue edition. Lanham, MD: Jason Aronson.

Kleiman, Tali, and Ran R. Hassin. 2011. "Non-Conscious Goal Conflicts." *Journal of Experimental Social Psychology* 47 (3): 521–532. doi:10.1016/j.jesp.2011.02.007.

Klein, Melanie. (1921) 2002. "The Development of a Child." In *Love, Guilt and Reparation and Other Works 1921–1945*. New York: Simon and Schuster.

McClelland, David C., Richard Koestner, and Joel Weinberger. 1989. "How Do Self-Attributed and Implicit Motives Differ?" *Psychological Review* 96 (4): 690–702. doi:10.1037/0033-295X.96.4.690.

Melnikoff, David E., Robert Lambert, and John A. Bargh. 2020. "Attitudes as Prepared Reflexes." *Journal of Experimental Social Psychology* 88 (May): 103950. doi:10.1016/j.jesp.2019.103950.

Molden, Daniel, and Angela Lee. 2008. "Motivations for Promotion and Prevention." In *Handbook of Motivation Science*, edited by James Y. Shah and Wendi L. Gardner, 169–187. New York: Guilford Press.

Reich, Wilhelm. 1925. *Der triebhafte Character: Eine psychoanalytische Studie zur Pathologie des Ich*. Leipzig: Internationaler Psychoanalysticher Verlag.

Shedler, Jonathan, Martin Mayman, and Melvin Manis. 1993. "The Illusion of Mental Health." *American Psychologist* 48 (11): 1117–1131. doi:10.1037/0003-066X.48.11.1117.

Smith, Adam. (1776) 1852. *An Inquiry into Nature and Causes of the Wealth of Nations*. London: T. Nelson.

Sommer, Kristin L., and Frank Bernieri. 2015. "Minimizing the Pain and Probability of Rejection: Evidence for Relational Distancing and Proximity Seeking Within Face-to-Face Interactions." *Social Psychological and Personality Science* 6 (2): 131–139. doi:10.1177/1948550614549384.

Wilson, Timothy D. 2004. *Strangers to Ourselves*. Cambridge, MA: Harvard University Press.

5 Nonlinear Multidimensional Language

In this chapter, we will shift the focus to communication strategies targeting unconscious thought. This could be a little difficult to envision at first since the aim is to understand a form of language that goes beyond conscious capabilities. Looking for a place to start with this ethereal subject matter, we return to Freud, who was instrumental in challenging society's belief that speech has only one true meaning.

In his 1901 book, *The Psychopathology of Everyday Life*, Freud described the potential meaningfulness of a large number of seemingly trivial or nonsensical, even bizarre, errors and slips of the tongue (parapraxis) (Freud and Gay, 1901). Freud believed that these errors in speech, memory, or physical action represent unconscious needs, wishes, or trains of thought obscured from conscious awareness.

In one of his examples, Freud recounts an instance when a woman speaking at a social gathering unconsciously expressed her sexual interests by announcing, "Yes, a woman must be pretty if she is to please the men. A man is much better off. As long as he has five straight limbs, he needs no more!" (Freud and Gay, 1901). This was not an attempt at locker-room humor. She had intended to say "four strong limbs."

I witnessed a similar slip while out hiking with my teenage son. It was hot so he removed his shirt, revealing tan skin and a large muscular chest. In his hand he held a long straight tree limb that he was using as a hiking pole. While passing other hikers, one starry-eyed girl greeted him saying, "Nice stick." As she spoke, her friend looked at her in disbelief. To make sense of her friend's reaction, she "listened" to her own statement and suddenly heard the rhyme. This was obvious because her face blushed, she turned her eyes to the ground (exposure shame), and quickly shuffled off down the trail while her girlfriend tried to conceal her laughter. I mention this contemporary example to make the point that slips of the tongue are not an archaic Victorian artifact.

This brings us to a fascinating figure in the field of psychoanalysis, Sandor Ferenczi (1873–1933), who was one of the earliest to argue that psychotherapy is a collaborative, mutually beneficial process in which the therapist and patient co-create reality. Most important, Ferenczi noticed that certain types of speech

DOI: 10.4324/9781003127208-5

are more likely to convey unconscious content, such as metaphors and analogies.

Ferenczi (1915) explained that,

> Sometimes one suspects something important behind an apparently haphazard choice of metaphor ... "A difficult birth," said one patient mockingly, as the analysis made no progress. He was unaware that the choice of this expression was determined by the difficult labor from which his own wife had suffered. On account of this difficult birth he could not hope for offspring, although meantime his first-born had died.
>
> (399)

Ferenczi (1915, 109) believed there was a special form of communication, which he termed "a dialogue of unconsciouses", in which "the unconscious of two people completely understand themselves and each other, without the remotest conception of this on the part of the consciousness of the other." This is due in part to the unique processing capabilities of unconscious awareness.

Twenty-five years later, while commenting on the pervasiveness of unconscious communication, Milton Erickson (1940) wrote, "as in dreams, puns, elisions, plays on words, and similar tricks that we ordinarily think of as frivolous—all play a surprising and somewhat disconcerting role in the communication of important and serious feelings" (Erickson and Kubie, 1940, 61). Here Erickson points not only to the fact that speech has multiple levels of meaning but also that unconscious processes may speak a different language.

Similarly, James (1890) observed that, "Men, taken historically, reason by analogy long before they have learned to reason by abstract characters" (vol. 2, 363). In addition to pointing to the unconscious origins of thought, James (1890) also points out that in all ancient oratory, "We find persuasion carried on exclusively by parables and similes" (vol. 2, 363). James also believed that stories are crucial to the growth of new knowledge.

This is the type of language most likely to mediate unconscious thought. The vocabulary of unconscious processes includes analogies, metaphors, stories/parables, homonyms, jokes, puns, and symbols or icons. It is the vernacular of dreams, poetry, and works of literary genius—a form of language that is expansive, nonlinear, and multidimensional.

Summarizing contemporary research on the nature of unconscious intelligence, Pawel Lewicki and colleagues (1992) report:

> A considerable amount of evidence indicates that as compared to consciously controlled cognition, the unconscious information-acquisition processes are incomparably faster and structurally more sophisticated. They allow for the development of procedural knowledge that is "unknown" to conscious awareness not merely because it has been encoded (and entered the memory system) through channels that are independent from consciousness. This knowledge is fundamentally

inaccessible to the consciousness because it involves a more advanced and structurally more complex organization than what could be handled by consciously controlled thinking.

(14)

In other words, conscious awareness is incapable of comprehending all that is known at unconscious levels.

Using the terminology of neuropsychology, we can think of communication in terms of signal processing. At conscious and unconscious levels, awareness focuses on analyzing (e.g., categorizing), modifying (e.g., gestalt completion), and synthesizing (e.g., inference) signals, such as sounds, images, and existing mental representations.

At the level of conscious awareness, the process is orderly, sequential, and linear. This awareness is made concrete in the form of rule-governed coding, such as math, logic, and formal syntax. But when we start examining the meaning of dreams, parables, and metaphors, more seems to be known than is consciously realized.

At unconscious levels, signals are processed in a manner that is nonlinear and multidimensional. This allows us to "know things" without knowing how we know. When put to conscious analysis, the complexity seems chaotic because the rules cannot be discerned. As stated by the philosopher, Gottfried Leibniz, 1686, "Quand une regle est fort composée, ce qui luy est conforme, passe pour irrégulier" (When a rule is extremely complex, that which conforms to it appears to be random).

As demonstrated in mathematics, nonlinear systems cannot be treated as linear systems, because nonlinear systems have chaotic behavior (multiple rules operating in tandem) and bifurcation (one item can split into multiple meanings). Most importantly, nonlinear systems do not have a canonical representation (universal meaning). An absence of canonical representation is most evident in the language of subjective reality, in which meanings are peculiar (based on the experience of a single individual) rather than normative. For example, when a person who is Catholic looks at a cross, that symbol will have certain unconscious meanings. But when a person who is Islamic looks at a cross, a different implicit meaning is produced. Thus, there can be no such thing as a dictionary of dream symbols or phallic symbols, because there is no universal meaning for objects processed at unconscious levels.

When considering unconscious communication, hypnotherapists often speak to a dissociated unconscious mind while using hypnotic language to influence its activities. But this hierarchical, unilateral approach to communication (an authority figure directing the patient) runs contrary to the egalitarian, collaborative, and co-creative principles of modern process work.

This brings us to one of the greatest contributions to hypnosis by Milton Erickson (1955), which was his concept of permissive suggestion. This open-ended method of suggestion was designed by Erickson to promote self-organizing change. In this model, hypnotherapeutic language merely serves as a catalyst for deep inner processing (self-directed problem solving). Metaphorically describing his approach, Erickson explains, "There is nothing more delightful than planting flower seeds and not knowing what kinds of flowers are going to come up" (Erickson and Rossi, 1979, 389). This type of growth-oriented, intrapsychic evolution is what characterizes all forms of psychotherapeutic process work at any level of consciousness.

5.1 Vocabulary Facilitates Thought

While reflecting on the ways in which education is connected to the care of human consciousness, William James (1916) argued that we problem solve more effectively when we have a vocabulary that allows us to clearly define the issue that confronts us. As James (1916, 116) explains, "The more adequate the stock of ideas, the more 'able' is a man, the more uniformly appropriate is his behavior likely to be." In other words, when equipped with a psychologically sophisticated vocabulary, people are better able to assess a situation and organize their response.

James then describes a less capable state of mind, one that is likely to leave an individual feeling either helpless or angry at the outside forces that seem to dictate his fate. According to James (1916, 116), "He who has few names is … an incompetent deliberator. The names—and each name stands for a conception or idea—are our instruments for handling our problems and solving our dilemmas." Thus, we use words as tools to help construct our thoughts as we problem solve.

Subsequently, modern research has shown that a psychometric tool, such as the Minnesota Multiphasic Personality Inventory (MMPI), can be used as a form of therapeutic assessment in which a test feedback session yields a reduction in symptomatic distress, a significant increase in self-esteem, and increased feelings of hope (Finn and Tonsager, 1992). The way this outcome is achieved is by empowering clients to frame their own assessment questions and soliciting their involvement in interpreting test results.

For example, the question might be asked, "Which of these descriptors seems most meaningful to you? How does it help you better understand your experience?" As argued by Finn and Martin (1997), this collaborative approach produces a psychoeducational opportunity during which the diagnostic profiles help enrich the client's introspective vocabulary. This new psychological vocabulary then informs clients' efforts to manage internal processes.

To help us think about this, we can go back to the insights of the brilliant developmental psychologist Lev Vygotsky (1896–1934), who observed that as thought and language emerge in childhood, children talk to themselves out loud as they problem solve. Vygotsky reasoned that by talking to themselves (self talk), children learn to guide and direct their own behaviors through difficult tasks and complex maneuvers.

This *self talk* later turns into an inner dialogue used by older children and adults to guide physical action, emotional reactions, and cognitive activity. Internalized self talk becomes highly complex and may take on positive or negative forms, such as encouraging one's self and listing important steps in a problem-solving sequence, or criticizing one's self and predicting failure. In all cases, the impact of self talk on behavior is substantial and somewhat dependent on the individual's vocabulary. Like the Jamesian pragmatic view of vocabulary, Vygotsky argues that our thoughts are realized in the words we use. As Vygotsky (1934, 251) puts it, "Experience teaches us that thought does not express itself in words, but rather realizes itself in them."

Currently, almost everyone agrees that language assists with conscious thought and discernment. Vygotsky (1978, 32) stated it poignantly when he wrote, "The child begins to perceive the world not only through his eyes but also through his speech." But what about implicit working memory and the goals it seeks to promote? Is it possible that self talk can occur unconsciously? If so, is there a special vocabulary that is better suited to the nonlinear, multidimensional nature of unconscious thought?

Consider the story of Bill W., a lifelong alcoholic whose physician, William D. Silkworth, described his condition as hopeless. Shortly after, Ebby T. handed Bill a copy of William James's *Varieties of Religious Experience*. His response was instantaneous and dramatic. As Bill explains,

> All at once I found myself crying out, "If there is a God, let Him show Himself! I am ready to do anything, anything!" Suddenly the room lit up with a great white light. I was caught up into an ecstasy which there are not words to describe. It seemed to me, in the mind's eye, that I was on a mountain and that a wind not of air but of spirit was blowing. And then it burst upon me that I was a free man. Slowly the ecstasy subsided. I lay on the bed, but now for a time I was in another world, a new world of consciousness.
>
> (cited in Lovern, 1985, 374–375)

James's book is rich in metaphor and symbolism, and it is filled with powerful stories written in poetic verse. Discovering a path to recovery, Bill W. went on to help found the world's first and most successful self-help group, Alcoholics Anonymous (AA).

I have not personally experienced something so profound, though I did have the distinct sensation of a light turning on in my mind after I read Milton Erickson's *My Voice Will Go With You* (Milton and Rosen, 1982). Similar to James's *Varieties*, Erickson's book is filled with compelling stories of people seeking help and overcoming seemingly insurmountable problems. Erickson uses a great deal of metaphor as the reader learns about formative events in his childhood or witnesses provocative exchanges between Erickson and his clients.

Halfway through the book, I realized that something was changing in me—something outside of conscious awareness. The emotional weight I had carried since adolescence was lifting. Without knowing why, I decided that I needed to stop reading—so as not to disrupt whatever my unconscious needed time to process.

Then, two weeks later, I felt ready to resume my reading. By the end, I had a distinct feeling of increased self-confidence, though I could not say why. I do not imagine the book "had a message I needed to hear"; rather, it helped enrich the vocabulary used by unconscious thought.

Another example of literature rich in metaphor producing beneficial effects comes from British hospitals during WWI. For veteran soldiers diagnosed with shell shock and/or morbid depression, the most effective known treatment was a nurse sitting at the bedside reading Jane Austen novels. David Owen (2016) suggested that Austen's provincial stories produced this effect by addressing the issue of war in ways that are submerged, indirect, and therefore subliminal.

Based on reports from clinical practice that stretch back as far as the late 1800s, an argument can be made for a system of language that has greater resonance with unconscious processes. And, when utilized in therapy, it seems to help clients find clarity in a way that they cannot consciously explain. In the following sections we will focus on linguistic devices commonly used by clinicians who practice either depth psychology or hypnotherapy—two branches from the same tree. While this is not an exhaustive list (it does not include the profound impact of facial expression, movement, gesture, and spatial distances), it "starts the ball rolling."

5.2 Metaphors and Analogies

George Lakoff and Mark Johnson (1980a; 1980b) reasoned that the human conceptual system is fundamentally metaphorical in character. Their point was that we can hardly think without access to metaphors, because they are how categories are understood, defined, and linked to other categories, even in concrete terminology.

As an example, think about the nominal category *heads of state*. We know implicitly what this means. A headless body cannot last long. Similarly, if a book is uplifting, we know that is good. If the stock market crashes, we know that is bad. It seems that gravity's effect on our bodies is a universal standard that structures abstract phenomena—vertically. Good is up (light hearted, on top of things) and bad is down (sinking spirits, being run into the ground).

The presence (or absence) of sunshine provides another standard. Thus, luminosity adds a double meaning to verticality: the *enlightenment* of *higher* education versus the *dim*wittedness of a *low* IQ; or heavenly light versus hell's darkness. These implicit meanings inform unconscious logic. Thus, *a fitting metaphor facilitates unconscious processing, just as words facilitate conscious deliberation.*

Lakoff and Johnson (1980a; 1980b) make the argument that because humans are physical beings moving in a world of physical objects, this (implicit) experiential learning shapes and constrains our thinking and understanding of reality. Or, as stated by William James (1912, 185, "reality is just what we feel it to be."

This leads to the argument that all language and meaning are embodied in the sense that concepts and cognitive processes are related to bodily experiences that occur while interacting with the environment. Because we are not able to consciously consider a lifetime of learning and unconscious perception, implicit metaphoric knowledge will always operate outside of (or prior to) conscious rationalized meaning. As Lakoff and Johnson explain, metaphoric meaning is subtextual, the foundation of understanding on which our abstract representations are constructed.

More than rhetoric, it seems that metaphors serve as a guide to new understandings. As stated in *conceptual metaphor theory*, the metaphorical structuring of meaning moves from embodied experience to a new domain of reasoning that is more abstract (where physical experience is lacking). According to philosopher Max Black (1962), a good metaphor is one that establishes a richer perspective on an uncertain object until increased familiarity causes the metaphor to become the object and, by doing so, cease to be metaphorical. For example, when we say that we are running late, we no longer think of it as a metaphorical description.

Bringing this discussion back to the therapeutic endeavor, it becomes apparent that any attempt at effective communication or reflective thought without the use of metaphor is woefully inadequate. It would be like trying to navigate a forest without having any access to maps or distinguishing landmarks. Metaphorical reasoning is an implicit vocabulary grounded in bodily experience, which helps unite reason and imagination. As Lakoff and Johnson (1980a) state,

> Reason, at the very least, involves categorization, entailment, and inference. Imagination, in one of its many aspects, involves seeing one kind of thing in terms of another kind of thing—what we have called metaphorical thought. Metaphor is thus *imaginative rationality*.
>
> (193; italics in original)

The use of imaginative rationality seems to impact the body. A client told a colleague that he was "sickened" by his newly recovered feelings. Subsequently, he became ill and was confined to his bed for two weeks. Thus, references to embodied experience, even when stated as an analogy, might be instrumental in understanding how to work with the peculiar (singular) logic of unconscious reason.

For example, a woman came to me and requested hypnosis for help with migraine headaches. They were so severe that she was unable to function at work. As she put it, "These migraine headaches leave me *flat on my back*." Therefore, I taught her self-hypnosis, told her to use it at the first sign of an approaching migraine, and told her to do it while lying *flat on her back*. The conscious logic, which I also offered, was that the position would help decrease the tension in her neck and increase blood flow.

She performed this exercise with enthusiasm. I was surprised by how much she loved her new floor hypnosis technique. She reported that it helped her avert the severe headaches, with an 85% reduction in overall pain. The technique seems to have fit her implicit understanding of the problem. I doubt that for anyone else it would have worked so well.

Moving to the literary meaning of analogies, we recognize that an analogy is comparable to metaphor in that it shows how two different things are similar. But, in literary works, analogies are often more cognitively complex and involve elements of logic that elicit both conscious and unconscious processing.

As a thought experiment, think of the psychological effect of *analogies being like the use of a sail and a rudder*—both are used simultaneously to navigate, but the sail acts on one resource (wind) while the rudder acts on another (water).

What was the effect of this sentence? Did your conscious mind examine the logic? Did your unconscious automatically connect this metaphor with the metaphor of the iceberg to maintain consistency (unconscious = underwater)? If you automatically assumed that the sail represented an unconscious domain (in the air) and the rudder represented a conscious domain (underwater), I would be surprised. The mind seeks familiarity and consistency.

Next, consider what happens when I tell you, "Say the first thing that comes to mind!" If you are a student of psychotherapy, the instant reply is either "Freud" or "free association." That is because analogies are a product of the associative knowledge that informs all automatic, unconscious processing. This identification of implicit connections is the psychotherapeutic version of analogy, which is near instantaneous and aimed almost exclusively at unconscious knowledge.

When a client, struggling to make progress, asks me, "Why can I not get past this sadness?" (as if I read minds), I can respond, "Say the first thing that comes to mind." A typical response is, "Well, the first thing that came into my mind is 'mother.' But that doesn't make sense, because she is a very loving mother." Whenever a client refers to a label for a parent (loving mother) or a spouse (good husband) as a substitute for actual behavior, know that things may not be as they seem.

A helpful follow-up question requests concrete details, such as saying, "Tell me about some of the loving things your mother does for you." Eventually, we will likely uncover some hurtful, passive-aggressive behavior or narcissistic self-justification or other well-disguised behavior by the mother. In this example, we end up with conscious process work, but it all begins with the unconscious vocabulary of analogy (my sadness = mother).

In a similar situation, I found myself using a single analogy to catalyze unconscious process work by saying, "Sometimes progress in therapy is a lot like being liberated." In this case, my client's parents had been holocaust survivors (that was why there were attachment issues during childhood). The use of this single term had a profound impact. Not only did she replace sadness with a feeling of enthusiasm, but she also stopped overeating. At a later session, she told me that my use of that word had deeply affected her though she could not say how or why (unconscious process work).

In general, we should recognize that analogies and metaphors are used to help structure knowledge of a new domain by carrying over the relations (experiential learning) from a known domain. In other words, they form an associative bridge. As a rule, familiar information is easier to process than novel information. Thus, during problem solving new problems are assumed to be analyzed based on their similarity to known problems. This is known as the *hermeneutic circle*, which is the principle that when seeking to learn something new, we start with what we already know. Thus, metaphors are not only figures of speech but instruments of knowing.

5.3 Narrative Transportation

If metaphors are the words of unconscious deliberation, then narratives extend imaginative rationality in the way that sentences extend the meaning of the words they contain (i.e., *stories are to metaphors as sentences are to words*). As an amalgamation of embodied experiences and emotional reactions, narratives serve as a multidimensional building block for the unconscious construction of meaning.

The effect of stories on consciousness has been studied in a model known as *narrative transportation theory*. Transportation is defined as an integrative melding of attention, imagery, and feelings focused on the story's events (Green and Brock, 2000). Researchers argue that stories compel the listener to "travel" or be mentally drawn into the reality described in a narrative as well as the outcomes associated with the narrative. By measuring the degree of transportation, researchers can predict the persuasive impact of narratives, with transported listeners frequently displaying increases in story-consistent beliefs, attitudes, and behaviors.

Using narrative transportation, therapists acquire the ability to simulate novel experiential realities rather than being limited to what the client is immediately perceiving and understanding or recalling from experience. Narrative transportation has also been found to influence central aspects of the mind, such as self-concept, and impact expectations for the future (Green and Sestir 2017). This makes story a particularly important therapeutic tool.

When done correctly, narrative transportation involves a strong sense of absorption. Like reading a compelling novel, transported listeners may experience vivid mental imagery and automatically identify with a main character.

To make our unconscious vocabulary rich, stories should not only contain quoted material but also some information on what the characters in the story were thinking, feeling, and hoping to achieve. Whenever possible, I use a story that will activate more than one feeling state. Like a good novel, an emotionally compelling story creates tears as well as laughter or fear as well as courage.

The absorptive effect is further enhanced by mentioning personal details (she had this warm smile, a lot like yours), situational factors (she also married before finishing college), and symptomatology that mimics client experiences (she had suffered from ten years of panic attacks, just a little longer than you). In any story about fellow human beings, there is always enough overlap that matching details will emerge. Because sincerity is keenly studied by unconscious perception, I stick to factual details when telling therapeutic stories.

With strong identification, the anecdotal evidence associated with other clients' positive outcomes will yield positive expectancy effects. If the client in the story improves, then the listener will implicitly expect a similar recovery.

Because I expect clients to automatically identify with the characters in my stories, I carefully focus on the extraordinary nature of these people, or I express compassion for their faults. Thus, when telling any story during therapy, even if it is a story about me or my family, I imagine that, for the client, I am telling a story about him or herself. Unconscious intelligence will be listening for predictions, suggestions, or associative primes. Figuratively speaking, all stories are about the individual who hears them. In therapy the story used to stimulate unconscious processing may literally be a story about the client (Chapter 7 will explore the stories we tell clients about themselves).

As a humous example, when a woman was struggling to assert herself with her mother, I told her that I had an inspiring story that I thought would help her. I then told her a story about another client of mine who had developed a very clever solution for managing her boss's demands. Then I confessed, "I am not entirely certain who told me this … I just remember really liking her solution."

My client was beaming. Bursting with pride, she raised her hand (I guess to help me identify her) and said, "That client was me!" I apologized for being so forgetful (I had only suspected it was her towards the end). However, she insisted that the story was exactly what she needed to hear. Sometimes, we need to learn about our own past by hearing the story told by others.

What Green and Clark's (2013) narrative transportation theory suggests is that individuals' cognitive, emotional, and imagery immersion in a narrative is a key mechanism of attitude, belief, and behavior change. In research into the same phenomena from a different perspective, it was discovered that people's implicit attitudes towards others can change nearly instantaneously when told an emotionally compelling story about that person.

For example, researchers Dessel, Ye, and Houwer (2018) instantly changed positive implicit attitudes towards Mahatma Gandhi after telling the alleged story of how Gandhi (due to religious reasons) refused the use of modern medicines on his sick wife. She died afterwards. But when Gandhi contracted the same illness shortly thereafter, he allowed the same treatment for himself and recovered. After hearing this, research subjects showed a more negative implicit attitude towards Gandhi. This research helps explain why gossip, in the form of storytelling, can be so insidious in its effects.

In therapy, if we recognize that unconscious semantics are more influenced by emotionally charged actions than by logical arguments, then we can mediate negative attitudes using the vocabulary of unconscious intelligence. Like the function of a sentence, narrative transportation integrates attention, feeling, and imagery at deep unconscious levels.

But just as sentences can be helpful or destructive, so too can a narrative. Whenever I tell a story, I am careful to consciously monitor each element of the story before saying it out loud. Always I ask myself, "Is this what the client needs to hear right now?" Occasionally, I catch some part of the story that is problematic and omit it from the narrative (subtraction). I can also enrich stories by sharing things that I wished would have happened (addition). For example, I might confess, "If I had known then what I know now, I could have told this person to do X, which would certainly have resulted in Y." Honest, creative reimagining is always better than resorting to dishonesty.

5.4 Externalization and Therapeutic Ambiguity

If narratives are to unconscious problem solving what sentences are to conscious logic, then I would argue that projectives (ambiguous objects) are the paper and pencil used to explore unconscious constructions. I will illustrate this concept with a story.

When my grandmother was dying of cancer, my mother was faced with an emotional challenge. My mother had lost her father to lung cancer when she was twelve, and her two-year-old child had been killed in a car accident. No doubt she was reminded of these tragic experiences as she cared for her dying mother.

Like any other person, my mother needed some means of integrating this emotionally destabilizing event into a forward-moving state of consciousness (everything will be okay). Hope and resiliency would be needed to protect her from the destructive urges that are sometimes triggered by the loss of a uniquely important attachment figure.

At a crucial moment, while sipping tea at my grandmother's house, my mother looked toward the horizon and saw a bright red cardinal perched in a tree. She thought to herself, "Wouldn't Grannie be pleased to see this."

Her mother, who was receiving palliative care at a hospice center, had always said that cardinals were a sign of good luck. Then, unexpectedly, the bird flew straight toward the house, landed on the patio, and peered through the glass door. My mother was captivated by the experience and could not wait to tell the story to her mother. What she did not know, consciously, was that this would be the same day that my grandmother breathed her final breath. For my mother, the cardinal was a sign from heaven that her mother would be in a better place surrounded by happiness.

What happens when we observe an isolated object that is not already linked to a causal chain of events? We automatically transform the object into a metaphor (inspiration) or a full-blown narrative (a sign). The more ambiguous the object, the more room for our unconscious to scribble out its constructions.

This fact was appreciated and further explored in the poetry of Justinus Kerner (1786–1862), and the private artwork of Victor Hugo (1802–1862). Both used ink blots to inspire their literary works and reconcile themselves with emotionally troubling events. The effect was powerful. In 1863, Hugo said of his *Tache* (stain) paintings, "These scribbles are for private use and to indulge very close friends" ("Ces griffonnages sont pour l'intimité et l'indulgence des amis tout proches.") (Hugo, 1909, 175). This psychological exercise became a popular parlor game named *Blotto*.

Seeing its psychological value, Hermann Rorschach (1884–1922) transformed the game into the Rorschach Ink Blot test. In doing so, he replaced supernatural explanations (communication with spirits or the dead) with a psychoanalytic understanding of unconscious mental activity.

The contemporary theory is that because projective techniques, such as ink blots, do not depend on higher levels of language development and conceptual understanding, the response they elicit is more likely a product of an implicit experiential system (imaginative rationalization), especially when the response is immediate and emotionally charged.

As an example, while still a doctoral intern, I was asked to administer the Rorschach Ink Blot test to a 14-year-old male. As expected, he saw the "bat" on the card that most people identify as being a bat. Then he got a card that could be interpreted as two women kissing (though many see it as two women singing). After that, the automatic, emotional processing really engaged. The next card was "women's breasts." The card after that was "two people having sex." And then, when we got to the more complex and stimulating ink blots, the boy suddenly covered his eyes, turned his chair to face away from me, and pleaded, "Why are you making me look at all of these dirty pictures?!"

After I described his reaction to my supervisor, she laughed and conjectured, "He must be starting puberty. He is developing strong sexual feelings and does not know what to do with them." Whether or not her interpretation was correct, the exercise helped me appreciate the active role unconscious processes play in shaping conscious perceptual experience.

All objects seen and sounds heard can have many possible interpretations and configurations within consciousness. Herman von Helmholtz (1821–1894) was the first to describe the role of imagination in all acts of visual perception—a theory of completion (Gregory, 1997) that led to the Gestalt emphasis on internal factors that help construct people's perceptions. Later those ideas were incorporated into Jerome Bruner's "New Look" psychology (1957), which challenged psychologists to study not just an organism's response to a stimulus, but also its internal interpretation—the role of implicit expectations in perception.

Much of the research done to support the New Look movement showed that unconscious expectations serve to resolve ambiguity (externalization). As defined by Jean Piaget (1896–1980), externalization is a process by which we attribute to things in the external world the products of our own mental activity. According to David Elkind (1976), this attribution is immediate, unconscious, and instrumental in establishing a fluid sense of reality.

Evidence from various corners of the cognitive sciences (using paradigms such as surprised cued recall, probe recognition, lexical decision, eye tracking, and cognitive load) suggests that the human mind makes causal inferences, predictions, and analyses of intentions automatically and largely unconsciously. Ran Hassin (2013) even argued that we can unconsciously conduct multiple inferences concurrently. Our task at present is to determine the most effective means of applying these powerful processing capabilities towards therapeutic ends.

In psychiatry, if you say that a disorder is *idiosyntonic*, it means that the patient is not personally suffering from the disorder because there is an inner resonance with the symptoms. This term seems to have evolved from Freud's (1914) use of the word ego-*syntonic* to describe pathological narcissism.

Because the word *idiosyntonic* literally means "a perfect fit for self," it is equally well-suited to describe any intervention that has been tailored to conform to the unconscious needs of implicit operations. Thus, I use the term *idiosyntonic suggestion* to describe an approach to self-suggestion that is derived from near instantaneous unconscious process work.

If someone sees a *sign* and self-suggests "that bird means that everything is going to turn out fine," then that is idiosyntonic suggestion. Because the choice is not forced and the conclusions are entirely spontaneous, the suggestion will be a perfect fit for the person.

When a person is asked to write down several words at random and then organize them into a sentence or a story (projective technique), the message that emerges will be a product of idiosyntonic suggestion. Not only does the ambiguity of several scattered words elicit externalization, the words are derived from unconscious associations to begin with. When a solution suddenly emerges, the therapeutic suggestion comes from the client's own unconscious intelligence.

Practically speaking, there are countless possibilities for creating therapeutic ambiguity. Here we will discuss four methods: *signs, projectives, ambiguous function assignments*, and *blank spaces*. While all of these elicit externalization, there are important differences:

- *Signs* are chance encounters with something unexpected (typically outside the office).
- *Projectives* are structured encounters with an ambiguous object (typically inside the office).
- *Ambiguous function assignments* (AFA) are open-ended tasks that do not have a clear objective.
- *Blank spaces* occur when the absence of sensory input becomes salient.

For example, if during a walk a client suddenly sees something meaningful in the clouds, that is a sign. If during therapy the client is handed a picture of clouds and asked what he sees, that is a projective. If without saying why the client is given the homework assignment of hiking to the top of a hill and lying down to watch the clouds, that is an AFA. If the client asks the therapist, "What do you think I should see in the picture of the clouds?"; the therapist suggests, "Close your eyes and see what comes to mind"; and the therapist then makes no further sound, that is the use of blank space. Any of these four can serve as "paper and pencil" for the expression of unconscious intelligence.

To promote process work outside the consultation room, I will tell clients to watch for signs. For example, "As you look for ways to deal with this tragedy in your past, pay attention to things going on around you. It is highly likely that you will see a sign, and this could be really important to you." Once after I said this to a client (who had been sadistically abused as a child), he came back two weeks later in a transformed state of mind. His anger and depression had vanished. He was smiling and telling me that for the first time he had experienced joy while interacting with his wife. I asked what had caused this dramatic shift, he replied,

> It happened on the way home from work, shortly after our last visit. As I drove down the highway, I looked to the West and saw that the sunset was going to be spectacular. I pulled over to the side of the road so that I could look at it. The sight was so beautiful! It caused me to burst into tears. I had never noticed beauty like this before. I took it as a sign that there can be goodness in my life.

When using projectives for process work, I employ a variety of objects, such as artwork on the wall, book titles on a bookshelf, symbolic images in a deck of cards, or automatic writing produced by the client. For example, with a client who felt unable to describe his problem, I gave him a piece of paper and told him to draw it. His dark, chaotic sketch opened a doorway to a complex and traumatizing past.

For another client, I tore a piece of paper into small pieces and had him write the first sixteen words that came to mind—each word on a separate piece. I then had him pick the most important words—ones that made his gut stir—and had him place them in order as a sentence. The sentence "told him" he hated his marriage because he had surrendered all personal power to his wife.

I do not offer any interpretations while working with projectives because conscious insight is not the goal. The primary objective is to engage unconscious intelligence in the process of defining the problem and constructing creative solutions. From this activity, important idiosyntonic suggestions will emerge.

Regarding AFAs, I have listened to other therapists describe strange rituals or even ordeals that clients are sent to perform, such as carrying a brick up a hillside. Allegedly, this works out well. However, my approach is to refrain from telling others to do something that I would not wish to do myself. So, if I use an ambiguous assignment, the action will be subtle, semi-purposeful, or enjoyable.

For example, a client might ask, "Is there anything I should be doing between sessions?" My response might be, "Yes. At some point during the week, surprise yourself." For one woman, who spent too much time alone in her apartment, I said, "If at any point during the week you feel your body wanting to go in a certain direction, follow the urge and see where it leads you." This assignment led her to her car and then to another town, where she treated herself to strawberry pie. Sitting in the homespun café that she had discovered, she suddenly realized how trapped she felt in Phoenix. Soon after, she quit her job and moved to Oregon, where she felt more at home.

Lastly, I believe that blank space (stimulus deprivation) is incredibly important for unconscious processing. I have seen profound results occur following a well-timed moment of silence during therapy. At a minimum, it is helpful for a therapist to slow down the back and forth of conversation so that brief moments of silence are afforded.

In some instances, when clients seem to be tripping over their words, I recommend a pause—a couple of seconds—between sentences. Or, I might have the client close his eyes and speak slowly. The change in cognition and emotionality is often surprising. In some instances, repressed memories or suppressed fears suddenly come thundering into conscious awareness.

With just a little bit of blank space, superficiality of thought is replaced with powerful realizations. In one such instance, when I told my client to slow down her speech, close her eyes, and breathe more deeply, she shifted to a conversation about her beloved father and suppressed fears that he would not accept her fiancée because it was an interracial relationship. The urgency of this awareness was not known to her consciously. A more subtle blank space is the unstated content that exists between one idea and another. I call these "gap thoughts" because they manifest as a gap in a conscious train of thought.

Anytime I hear a client unexpectedly switch to a new topic without a clear transitional statement, I focus the client's attention on the blank space. My assumption is that the gap contains latent associative structures.

For example, the other day while helping a woman, who was very upset with her husband (no longer speaking to him), I noticed that she suddenly transitioned to remarks about her biological mother (who had been extremely abusive). Wishing to explore this blank space, I asked her, "What caused you to go from talking about your husband not doing enough to help you with your pregnancy to a discussion about your biological mother?"

With tears forming in her eyes, she revealed (to me and to herself),

> When I said that he is a good father (to her son from a previous marriage) … and I know he will be a good father to our new daughter—I think it made me wonder if I will know how to form a mother-daughter relationship … with a girl. Child protective services put me in an orphanage because my mother was so abusive.

She could not say anything else beyond that because of emotional flooding. But now equipped with better understanding, I was able to provide helpful suggestions and predictions about her future as a mother. Once she no longer felt so poorly about herself (an unconscious fear that she will replicate her mother's parenting) and with the threat of failure reduced, her anger at her husband evaporated. The following week she had nothing but kind words to say about him. It seems that her anger had been displaced.

In this case example, and most others listed in this book, you can find instances of conscious process work blended in with unconscious process work. We identify a reaction as conscious process work whenever a person "realizes" something important. By contrast, unconscious processing does not always lead to conscious insight. Much of our perception, memory, learning, and motivation (i.e., problem-solving) is implicit and therefore not governed by conscious oversight. This is why I consider unconscious processing to be of primary importance to the therapeutic endeavor. To be clear, I am not making the argument that conscious insight is unnecessary; rather, I do not believe it is sufficient.

Chapter 5 Key Points

- Unconscious knowledge is largely inaccessible to conscious intelligence because it involves a more advanced, structurally complex organization than what can be consciously processed.
- A rich vocabulary is essential to mental problem-solving. Furthermore, unconscious intelligence works best with its own multidimensional, nonlinear vocabulary.
- Metaphors and analogies are not only figures of speech but instruments of knowing.
- Stories are an elaboration of metaphorical meaning that can facilitate unconscious learning by conveying novel experiential realities.
- Therapeutic ambiguity (signs, projectives, AFA, blank spaces) helps represent the piecemeal products of unconscious intelligence as it works out its solutions.

References

Black, Max. (1962) 2019. *Models and Metaphors: Studies in Language and Philosophy*. Ithaca, NY: Cornell University Press.

Bruner, Jerome S. 1957. "On Perceptual Readiness." *Psychological Review* 64 (2): 123–152. doi:10.1037/h0043805.

Dessel, Pieter Van, Yang Ye, and Jan De Houwer. 2018. "Changing Deep-Rooted Implicit Evaluation in the Blink of an Eye: Negative Verbal Information Shifts Automatic Liking of Gandhi." *Social Psychological and Personality Science* 10 (2): 266–273. doi:10.1177/1948550617752064.

Elkind, David. 1976. *Child Development and Education: A Piagetian Perspective*. Oxford: Oxford University Press.

Erickson, Milton H. 1955. "Self-Exploration in the Hypnotic State." *Journal of Clinical and Experimental Hypnosis* 3 (1): 49–57. doi:10.1080/00207145508410131.

Erickson, Milton H., and Lawrence S. Kubie. 1940. "The Translation of the Cryptic Automatic Writing of One Hypnotic Subject by Another in a Trance-Like Dissociated State." *The Psychoanalytic Quarterly* 9 (1): 51–63. doi:10.1080/21674086.1940.11925407.

Erickson, Milton H., and Sidney Rosen. 1982. *My Voice Will Go With You: The Teaching Tales of Milton H. Erickson, MD.* New York: W. W. Norton & Company.

Erickson, Milton H., and Ernest L. Rossi. 1979. *Hypnotherapy: An Exploratory Casebook.* Har/Cas edition. New York: Irvington Pub.

Ferenczi, Sandor. (1915) 2019. *Further Contributions to the Theory and Technique of Psycho-Analysis.* London: Routledge.

Finn, Stephen E., and Hale Martin. 1997. "Therapeutic Assessment with the MMPI-2 in Managed Health Care." In *Personality Assessment in Managed Health Care: Using the MMPI-2 in Treatment Planning*, edited by J. N. Butcher, 131–152. New York: Oxford University Press.

Finn, Stephen E., and Mary E. Tonsager. 1992. "Therapeutic Effects of Providing MMPI-2 Test Feedback to College Students Awaiting Therapy." *Psychological Assessment* 4 (3): 278–287. doi:10.1037/1040-3590.4.3.278.

Freud, Sigmund. 1914. "Zur Einführung Des Narzißmus." *Jahrbuch Für Psychoanalytische Und Psychopathologische Forschung* 6 (1): 1–24.

Freud, Sigmund, and Peter Gay. (1901) 1989. *The Psychopathology of Everyday Life.* Translated by James Strachey. New York: W. W. Norton & Company.

Green, Melanie C., and Timothy C. Brock. 2000. "The Role of Transportation in the Persuasiveness of Public Narratives." *Journal of Personality and Social Psychology* 79 (5): 701–721. doi:10.1037/0022-3514.79.5.701.

Green, Melanie C., and Jenna L. Clark. 2013. "Transportation into Narrative Worlds: Implications for Entertainment Media Influences on Tobacco Use." *Addiction* 108 (3): 477–484. doi:10.1111/j.1360-0443.2012.04088.x.

Green, Melanie C., and Marc Sestir. 2017. "Transportation Theory." In *The International Encyclopedia of Media Effects*, edited by P. Rössler, C. A. Hoffner, and L. Zoonen, 1–14. Malden, MA: John Wiley & Sons. doi:10.1002/9781118783764.wbieme0083.

Gregory, Richard L. 1997. "Knowledge in Perception and Illusion." *Philosophical Transactions: Biological Sciences* 352 (1358): 1121–1127.

Hassin, Ran. 2013. "Yes It Can." *Perspectives on Psychological Science: A Journal of the Association for Psychological Science* 8 (2): 195–207. doi:10.1177/1745691612460684.

Hugo, Victor. 1909. *Correspondence entre Victor Hugo et Paul Maurice*, edited by Jules Claretie. Paris: Bibliothèque-Charpentier. https://archive.org/details/correspondanceе00hugo/page/174/mode/2up.

James, William. (1890) 1927. *The Principles of Psychology*, Vol. I–II. New York: Henry Holt.

James, William. 1912. *Essays in Radical Empiricism.* Edited by Ralph Barton Perry. New York: Longmans, Green & Co. Project Gutenberg. http://www.gutenberg.org/ebooks/32547.

James, William. (1916) 1925. *Talks To Teachers On Psychology; And To Students On Some Of Life's Ideals.* New York: Henry Holt. Project Gutenberg. http://www.gutenberg.org/ebooks/16287.

Lakoff, George, and Mark Johnson. 1980a. *Metaphors We Live By.* Chicago: University of Chicago Press.

Lakoff, George, and Mark Johnson. 1980b. "The Metaphorical Structure of the Human Conceptual System." *Cognitive Science* 4 (2): 195–208.

Leibniz, Gottfried Wilhelm. (1686) 2012. *Discourse on Metaphysics and Other Writings*. Peterborough, ON: Broadview Press.

Lewicki, Pawel, Thomas Hill, and Maria Czyzewska. 1992. "Nonconscious Acquisition of Information." *American Psychologist* 47 (6): 796–801. doi:10.1037/0003-066X.47.6.796.

Lovern, J. D. 1985. "Unconscious Factors in Recovery from Alcoholism: The James-Jung-Erickson Connection." In *Ericksonian Psychotherapy, Vol. II: Clinical Applications*, edited by Jeffrey K. Zeig, 373–383. New York: Bruner/Mazel. Owen, David. 2016. "Conscripting Gentle Jane: Getting the Austen Treatment in the Great War." In *Writings of Persuasion and Dissonance in the Great War*, edited by David Owen and Maria Christina Pividori, 31–45. doi:10.1163/9789004314924_004.

Vygotsky, L. S. 1978. *Mind in Society: The Development of Higher Psychological Processes*. Cambridge, MA: Harvard University Press.

Vygotsky, Lev Semenovich. (1934) 2012. *Thought and Language*. Translated by Alex Kozulin. Cambridge, MA: MIT Press.

6 Prediction

While working at a setting filled with other professionals, a colleague noticed a woman leaving my office and later asked, "Where do you get such beautiful patients?" Jokingly, he added, "Can I pay you to refer her to me?" Not only was this woman exceptionally beautiful, she was also kind, charming, intellectually curious, and the owner of a successful business. She wanted my help to improve her skills as a mother—a single mother.

Despite outward appearances, this woman was in agony. During her private session, with tears running down her face, she asked, "Why does no man want to marry me? Why do men only use me and then leave me?" Not knowing what to say, I probed further, asking, "Have you never had a man propose to you?" In visible pain, she shook her head no.

After a moment of silence, I asked, "When did you first get the idea that no man will ever marry you?" After looking off to the side for a moment, she answered,

> I was nineteen. I was in a fight with my mother out by the garage. She was telling me that I am too rebellious. She was so angry. She said, "No man will ever want to marry a girl such as you!"

This prediction had shaped the course of her life, without any conscious awareness or intent.

How do you help a person caught in this type of mental trap? What tools does psychotherapy offer? The answer is obvious. But some of you will not like it. You have been taught not to trust the most straightforward solution—fighting fire with fire. The best way to counter a negative prediction is by offering a positive prediction.

The art of prediction predates recorded history, and yet it is as modern as artificial intelligence. Whether it is blessings versus curses or evolutionary algorithms, unconscious processes are readily influenced by predictions. These predictions not only influence conscious decisions and choices but also implicit expectancies that guide attention, motivation, action sequencing, and the formation of goals. Most importantly, predictions shape our emerging sense of self,

DOI: 10.4324/9781003127208-6

such as when a child goes to his father and asks, "What kind of man do you think I will grow up to be?"

It is not just parents who are called upon to predict the future. Socially sanctioned predictionists are embedded in every aspect of society: scientists forecast, doctors make prognoses, business leaders write annual forecasts, tournament organizers seed players, political pundits interpret polls, spiritual advisors receive revelations, and psychics tell fortunes. In contrast, a traditionally trained psychotherapist is likely to deflect questions of the future ("Tell me what you think will happen"). Almost every serious social enterprise has legitimized the act of making skillful predictions. While some psychotherapies offer stages of recovery or a hopeful prognosis for all members of human society, the incredible power of a convincing prediction can be used more strategically and with greater tailoring to the needs of the individual.

After reviewing *Consumer Reports* surveys, Scott Miller and Mark Hubble found that Americans rated psychics more helpful than therapists and were more likely to use their services. Miller and Hubble's (2017) explanation for this failure to meet consumer's needs is that the "secular constructions, reductionist explanations, and pedestrian techniques that so characterize modern clinical practice fall flat, failing to offer people the kinds of experiences, depth of meaning, and sense of connection they want in their lives" (Miller, 2017). One of the experiences that I believe people need is emotionally compelling predictions from a trusted authority.

For example, one day I had a client come to my office trembling, sobbing, and perseverating, "Oh my god! My husband is going to die and it's going to be all my fault! He's going to wake up, and it's going to kill him when he learns that I lost all the money!" After helping her recollect herself, my client explained that her husband was in a coma after suffering a massive heart attack. The doctor expected him to recover but warned my client, "Don't say anything to upset him. It could kill him." Her fear was that when her husband awoke from his coma, the first question would be, "Where did you put that large wad of cash that I was traveling with?"

He had suffered a heart attack while on vacation. After her husband had been flown by helicopter to the hospital, my client returned home with all their vacation cash. Frightened that someone would break in and steal the money, she hid it—as she said, "Where no one would ever find it."

When people set that goal for themselves, what they fail to realize is that the self-suggestion means that they will also be unable to find the item when they search for it. She had spent the previous seven days opening every drawer, searching every cupboard, unfolding every sheet, looking under the mattress—everywhere. She was exhausted and could not think of anywhere else to look. She cried, "Doc, you've got to help me! I can't make myself remember where I hid the money!"

I assured her that I would help her find the money and suggested that we use hypnosis. I spent approximately twenty minutes having her relive the series of events, including the moment she stashed the cash. When I told her to open her eyes and return to normal awareness, the first words out of her mouth were, "Doc, I got nothing! It didn't work! I got nothing!"

Not ready to give up, I asked, "Are you absolutely certain there is not any thought or image that came to mind … perhaps far away in the back of your mind?" She said, "Well, yes. I got 'the middle.' But I don't know the middle of what!" This was clearly a dead end.

Because the initial processing had not led to success, I assumed an incubation period would be required. This technique, which is characterized by the absence of conscious effort (conscious surrender), will be more fully explained in Chapter 9. After such an incubation period, a creative solution can suddenly emerge into consciousness without warning and, apparently, without effort.

I explained my expectations to her,

> The answer is inside of you. Sometimes it does not come out right away during hypnosis, but I am certain it will come to you within the next seven days while you are doing things around the house. But the answer will not be so straightforward. Instead, you will get a feeling that you should go somewhere, and it may not make much sense. The urge will probably come at an inconvenient time. You might be tempted to ignore it. But do not do that. You must follow the urge immediately, no matter where it leads you. Eventually your unconscious mind will take you to the money.

Her reply was, "I hope you're right. I know when he wakes up, the first thing he is going to want to know is what I did with the money."

Seven days later she returned to the office smiling. She was obviously pleased with herself and had found the money. She related,

> I did what you said. You told me to go home and stop thinking about it. So, I just started doing business as usual. Then one day I was watching TV. It was a show I used to watch with my husband. In the middle of my show, I got the thought, "I should take a shower." I thought that was really strange because I usually take my showers in the morning. But I remembered what you said, so I turned off the TV and went into my bedroom. But when I got there, I suddenly noticed my vanity table on the other side of my bedroom. I felt myself want to walk toward the vanity so I followed the feeling. It has two sets of drawers, one on each side. I found myself looking at the left side, at the middle drawer. That is where I keep all my stockings. I knew that I had already checked that drawer, and the money wasn't in there. But I went ahead and opened it. There I saw three rows of stockings. So, I reached for the middle row, right at the center. Then I squeezed the stocking and felt the money clip. Doctor Short, do you know what I did? I rolled the cash inside my stocking! I would have never found it.

Practitioners trained in hypnotherapy might identify this as an instance of post-hypnotic suggestion, though hypnosis formally ended before I made my prediction. The concept of post-hypnotic suggestion traces all the way back to Abbé Faria (1756–1819), who was the first healer to intentionally practice suggestion without the use of trance and the first to use post-hypnotic suggestion.

Using the language of the time to describe unconscious process work, Faria (1814) stated, "Nothing comes from the magnetizer; everything comes from the subject and takes place in his imagination; [it is] autosuggestion generated from within the mind [of the subject]" (Surbled, 1913, 605). What Faria demonstrated with experimentation was that if you predict that something will occur in the near future, unconscious imagination will produce these results. Thus, post-hypnotic suggestion is jargon for the use of prediction within a hypnotherapeutic context.

This was a crucial distinction that separated hypnotherapy from psychotherapy. Hypnotherapists remained willing to make predictions (following certain hypnotic rituals), whereas "non-directive" therapies rejected the practice.

While the strategic use of prediction is as old as antiquity, post-hypnotic suggestion is the clearest example of a clinical approach strategically eliciting prediction effects. However, there are some interesting differences between hypnotic suggestion and premodern forms of prediction.

Suggestion essentially moves the idea of personal agency from conscious effort to unconscious, automatic processes. For example, suggestions, such as "You will forget about your fear of rejection," create concrete response expectancies—a subjective probability that a response will occur and be experienced as automatic or non-volitional. As explained by Irving Kirsch (1990), who introduced this concept, these personal behaviors are experienced passively rather than feeling that we can produce them at will.

In contrast, premodern prediction moves agency away from the individual to outside forces, such as providence or ordained fate. For example, a fortune teller might proclaim, "It is your destiny to meet a mysterious man who will fall in love with you." Similarly, while reflecting on the influence of a prediction upon the event predicted, science philosopher Karl Popper (1977) uses the tragedy of *Oedipus* (who unwillingly fulfilled a prophecy that he would kill his father and marry his mother) to make the point that the oracle played the most important role in the sequence of events that led to the eventual outcome.

These *experiential expectancies* impact the way we act towards others by mitigating how we interpret their actions. A confirmatory bias causes us to perceive others in a light that favors the predicted behavior. As a person starts to interact differently with his or her environment, this influences others to reciprocate with complimentary behavior. The result is a self-fulfilling prophecy. Most importantly, these experiential expectancies for other people and events operate independently of the owner's efforts or intentions.

Because this form of prediction is not limited to the agency of the client, these predictions have greater flexibility than suggestion. As I said to a female client (who was horribly intimidated by male authority figures), "Within the next year your work will finally start to be appreciated. After that, your boss will offer you a promotion." The prediction undoubtedly primed certain behaviors without conscious awareness that she was acting differently. Although she did recognize that she was talking more casually with her boss about some of her struggles, she could not explain why he unexpectedly advanced her to "team-lead" on a very important project. One explanation is that the experiential expectancy (some force outside of me will make it happen) helped circumvent her performance anxiety and replaced it with leader-like confidence.

It is reasonable to predict that some readers will question the wisdom of making predictions when there is no way to ensure their fulfillment. What if the girl had not received any sort of promotion within a year's time? It is possible to botch predictions, but it is not likely if you are using common sense.

In this example, I was addressing a professional person who was obviously skillful, dedicated to hard work, and not already at the top of the organizational chart. In American industry, twelve months is the standard amount of time to at least be considered for a raise, if not some other more impressive promotion. So, the prediction is not much of a stretch. The outcome is placed in the remote future and the term "promotion" is vague enough to mean many different things, such as a raise or being put in charge of a project.

If I make a prediction that fails, then I always take the burden of failure on myself and move on to a new prediction. For example, I might say,

> I clearly misread the situation. Now that I have learned more about your work environment, I see that the promotions are only going to men and not deserving women, such as yourself. It is going to be difficult to stay at this job when there are other places out there that would recognize your talents.

The additional, common-sense prediction shifts attention from an experiential expectancy to a response expectancy. Thus, predictions can be worded in such a way as to target response expectancies or experiential expectancies. Either way, prediction is meant to bypass the limitations of conscious intention and engage unconscious problem solving and goal-oriented activity.

Keep in mind that most clients do not expect their therapist to be flawless. They just need someone to help them figure out how to move forward when they feel stuck or incapable. For problems that exceed the limits of conscious self-regulation, credible predictions help activate unconscious goal-oriented problem solving, which includes implicit experiential knowledge and persistence despite setbacks. The beauty of experiential expectancies is that it takes the pressure off. The benefit of response expectancies is that they lead individuals to believe in themselves.

Hypnotherapy clearly makes use of the latter form of prediction (response expectancies). In contrast, traditional process-oriented therapies, as well as cognitive therapies, have no such device. While Kirsch and colleagues (1995) have not formally studied the clinical benefits of *experiential expectancies* (the types of predictions often made by fortune tellers), it is interesting to note that their meta-analysis of studies showed that a therapy that does not incorporate prediction (cognitive behavioral) was out performed in at least 70% of the cases when hypnotherapy was added as a supplemental element.

6.1 Stacking Predictions

When making a prediction, it is helpful to think of a row of dominos. If the clinician uses multiple predictions in a stacked manner, then the fulfillment of one simple prediction starts a chain reaction. Along similar lines, Kirsch (1990) argued that the rationales accompanying treatments should not forecast too great an initial change. Kirsch believes it is better to create an expectation that *some* change in the desired direction will occur so that small fluctuations in the client's condition can be interpreted as evidence of progress.

Rather than making a single hard-to-believe prediction (e.g., you will meet the man of your dreams), it is better to stack predictions in a way that establishes progress markers. In this series, the realization of a more immediate prediction solidifies the expectations of each subsequent prediction. Stacked predictions function in the same way as setting a series of short-term goals that lead to the fulfillment of a long-term goal. The difference is that predictions activate goal-oriented pursuits without the need for conscious intention or conscious working memory (automatic behavior).

Returning to the case example with the missing cash, there were three important predictions in the stack:

1. Your unconscious will provide you with the information at home (spatial detail);
2. Your body will feel like walking in some direction (embodied experience); and
3. If you follow that feeling, you will locate the hidden money within the week (temporal detail).

Understand that the reason for this information is not to control behavior but instead to provide a target for goal-oriented processes operating outside of conscious awareness. As Kirsch (1990, 188) puts it, "The promise of improvement remoralizes patients and restores their faith in the future. Because hopelessness is a large part of what brought them into treatment, the restoration of hope constitutes a large part of the cure."

6.2 Spatial and/or Temporal Framing

While discussing post-hypnotic suggestions, Erickson stated, "*You present new ideas and new understandings, and you relate them in some undisputable way to the remote future*" (Erickson and Rossi, 1975, 148). New ideas lack relevancy until they are embodied and framed within experiential reality. The two most obvious frames for physical experience are time and space.

The prediction, "You will feel much stronger by your next birthday," is an example of temporal framing. Similarly, the prediction, "You will feel much better once you return home," is an example of spatial framing. In the case that was just mentioned, we see the use of spatial (it will happen at home) and temporal framing (at an inconvenient moment).

There are many instances of Erickson recommending a temporal frame that places life transforming events in the remote future, rather than something that is expected to happen soon. I had always wondered why. Then I saw research by Gilovich and colleagues (1993) indicating that people tend to feel more optimistic about a distal future (rather than a proximal future) because a distal future is represented more abstractly. In contrast, a proximal future event is viewed in greater concrete detail, thus there are more questions to be answered, which generates greater skepticism. In addition, studies show that when research participants thought about a distant problem, they came up with more possible solutions than when a problem fell closer to them in space or time (e.g., Trope and Liberman, 2010).

The frames that are created should be broad rather than narrow. If the structure is too tight, the person will feel trapped. If it is too loose, the person will not know where or when to expect the predicted event. Temporal framing can create an encapsulated space (no sooner than, no later than), as demonstrated by Erickson speaking to a young person who struggled with enuresis,

> Now, having a dry bed is a very difficult job. You might have your first dry bed in two weeks. And there has to be a lot of practice, starting and stopping. Some days you may forget to practice starting and stopping. That's all right. Your body will be good to you. It will always give you further opportunities. And some days you may be too busy to practice starting and stopping, but that's all right. Your body will always give you opportunities to start and stop. It would surprise me very much if you had a permanently dry bed within three months. It would also surprise me if you didn't have a permanently dry bed within six months. And the first dry bed will be much easier than two dry beds in succession. And three dry beds in succession is much harder. And four dry beds in succession is still harder. After that it gets easier. You can have five, six, seven, a whole week of dry beds. And then you can know that you can have one week of dry beds and another week of dry beds.
>
> (Erickson and Rosen, 1982, 11)

If worded correctly, the temporal frame associated with a prediction can also be stretched to cover a lifetime. I am likely to offer a reoccurring, positive prediction when resiliency is an important factor. This is achieved by priming hope, dedication, and a sense of purpose and then connecting these to a reoccurring event. A lifetime frame is illustrated in the next case example.

In this case, my client had suffered a tragic loss. She and her husband had been coming to me for marriage counseling, and it was working well. Their intimacy, trust, and deep affection for one another was rekindled. They decided to celebrate their marriage with a couple's getaway. But, on the first night, the husband died from an undetected heart condition.

His wife, who was now a single mother of three children, was engulfed in suicidal urges. Due to her own attempts to kill herself there in the hotel room, she had to be hospitalized. After being discharged from the hospital, a female therapist skillfully managed her individual care.

Eleven months later, she was faced with the one-year anniversary of her husband's death. Fearful that this could trigger the suicidal urges once again, she reasoned that she needed help from her couples therapist (me), because an anniversary is a couple's event. During therapy, I pointed out that throughout the year there are a great number of anniversaries that we experience, some negative, some positive. When I asked for her favorite anniversary, she said it was her birthday. I used this concept metaphorically as I discussed the proper way to celebrate the anniversary of a person's death.

This prime (a metaphorical juxtaposition of birth and death) would be too complex to process consciously. Logically, it makes no sense. But for unconscious intelligence, it is a problem-solving challenge to address using nonlinear, multidimensional logic.

Her first insight was that she did not want to be alone on this day. She wanted to surround herself with others who respected, admired, and loved her husband.

She asked me where the gathering should be hosted. So, I made my first prediction, "If you have this party in your home (spatial framing), it will help bring joy to the children and you." Next, I added some logic for her to consciously consider, "But even more importantly, it will be easier for you to remain in charge of what is happening since this is your home. You will be able to lead the group toward doing things that are meaningful to you." I was seeking to empower her because she had been struggling to assert herself within the extended family.

Together, we discussed possible group activities. The idea she liked most was for everyone to share their favorite memory of her husband and make a film of the replies for her to keep. My client wrote these ideas down and seemed eager to implement the plan. In other words, she was now looking forward to this potentially devastating anniversary date. Then I made the larger prediction, "I know for a fact that if you are able to embrace this first anniversary as a loving celebration, every year thereafter you will have nothing to worry about" (an *if/then* contingency combined with lifelong temporal framing).

As stated in TMT motivational theory, it seems that the perceived utility of a given mental representation increases exponentially as the deadline nears. In the case above, the woman's feelings and thoughts surrounding her husband's death needed to somehow be reorganized. The prime I indirectly established took the positively valenced values from one category of experience and bridged them to another: a "deathday" can be like a birthday. The closer she came to the anniversary date, the more powerfully the prime affected her. Later, she let me know that this celebration was one of the most meaningful that she had ever experienced.

In addition to motivation, issues of time and space must be considered when dealing with emotional reactions. Some predictions will intensify unconscious fears of failure if they are not allocated to some point in the remote future.

For example,

> I know you will find a man to marry and become a mother. You are not likely to reach menopause for another ten years at the very earliest. Given your current progress in therapy, it will take no more than five years for you to find the right man and marry him. Of course, it could happen before then, but five years at the latest.

This prediction was made for a woman who had spent the last ten years in unsuccessful relationships with men that either cheated on her or abandoned her. Her greatest fear was that she would never become a mother. Twelve months after my prediction she met someone who would be a good husband. After a year of dating, they married. Three years after that she gave birth to her first child (five years total).

In other cases, the need for change is urgent, so the prediction needs to focus on immediate events. For example,

SHORT: You are having panic attacks and feeling very fearful because your doctor said you may have some genetic disorder that could lead to heart attack. And you don't want to get tested because you are afraid that if the defective gene is there, you will be in constant fear. Is that right?

CLIENT: Yes! That doctor put me in a terrible predicament. I don't feel that I can get the test, and I don't feel that I cannot get the test. I wish I would have never gone to him.

SHORT: I just need to have you answer one question. And, after you answer that question, all your panic and fear will disappear. But before I ask my question, I need to know if you realize that you are mortal, that death is sort of unavoidable at some point.

CLIENT: Yes, I understand that.

SHORT: Then this is my question. Answer with the first thing that comes to mind. *What would be the best way to die?*

CLIENT: Massive cardiac arrest as I sleep.[Lots of blank space]

SHORT: Is there anything else we need to discuss? Do you need any other therapy?

CLIENT: No. I am fine now. I do not need to get the test. I have other things that I would rather be focusing on.

My prediction was for an outcome that would occur in less than a minute. Sometimes all that is needed is a few moments of unconscious processing.

6.3 Mysterious Means to a Certain End

My repeated experience has been that when I tell patients how to do something, it does not produce results that are as impressive as predicting it will occur. Especially when the prediction is stated in a way that stimulates an unconscious need to answer the question of *how to implement.*

For example, when confronted with their own limiting beliefs, clients will sometimes make a direct request for a prediction. A woman who has a history of staying in abusive relationships may ask, "Do you think I will ever have a boyfriend who is not a jerk?" To which I confidently respond, "I know that you will. I am certain of it. But neither you nor I can know exactly how this will occur."

This prediction is a prime, not a suggestion. I am predicting situational change but not suggesting any behavioral change. This causal ambiguity takes all the pressure off her, which is important if the person has a weak ego or low self-efficacy. The distinction is subtle but important. The type of prediction that elicits unconscious activity is ambiguous, which means it lacks details needed for conscious implementation. There is no plan for how to make it happen, just the assurance that it will happen.

If you are feeling doubtful that the technique of making predictions will have much impact on someone trained in critical thought, consider the following case. This 52-year-old client was an award-winning scientist who had worked as an experimental psychologist at the National Institutes of Health (NIH). He was a well-educated, rational thinker. Yet he could not escape the effects of a damning negative prediction.

It had only been a little over a year since his marriage had ended painfully. His wife first cheated on him, then divorced him, even as he was attempting to repair the marriage. She had convinced herself that she was the victim in this failed marriage, and now it was his turn to suffer. So, one day she called him with some important news.

She had been to see a psychic, and while there she asked about her husband's future. Allegedly, the psychic told her that he would die from colon cancer within five years. Even worse, he would be unable to remarry and therefore die alone.

The psychic then heralded dead spirits, allegedly establishing contact with my client's dead father. The father was a special person in my client's subjective world—someone who had always treated him and his mother with kindness. However, the psychic revealed that his father had deep, dark secrets, he had cheated on my client's mother, and he never really loved her. These revelations left my client in a state of psychological devastation and fear.

As he explained it to me,

> Dan, I don't believe in this bullshit. I don't think fortune telling is real. But I can't get it out of my head. Now I am terrified that I am going to die of colon cancer, alone! Even though I recently had a colonoscopy and everything was clear. It doesn't matter how much I tell myself that this garbage is not true … I am afraid that my unconscious might produce cancer as a result of a self-fulfilling prophecy! Can you use hypnosis or something to help me?

I told him that I did not think hypnosis was the best solution for this unique problem. My statement was, "Sometimes it's best to fight fire with fire." I then made a couple of predictions, "Your wife clearly went to a two-bit psychic who does not know what she is doing. Channeling the dead is a con artist ploy. None of her predictions will come true."

After thoroughly discrediting the source of the problematic primes, I made my second prediction,

> As luck would have it, I happen to know of an exceptionally skillful psychic who lives here in Phoenix. I have monitored her predictions with two other clients. Every single prediction she made came true. So, if you go to her, you will get a better take on your future.

His reply was, "Does it matter that I do not believe in psychics?" To which I replied, "You tell me. How much have you been affected by your wife's psychic, whom you have not actually met?" He saw the logic and took the number for "Brandi the Psychic."

I had confidence in Brandi's work, otherwise I would not have made the referral. She had phoned me in the past to seek consultation for a client who disclosed suicidal ideation. Brandi wanted to know what referrals to make and what resources to provide the young girl. Her actions were caring and responsible.

After his visit with Brandi, my client was psychologically transformed. She had predicted that he would live a long, active life. She also saw him meeting a wealthy business investor, soon, who would help him start a new business, which happened (the guy was a millionaire from Florida). She said within the year he would be dating someone whose beauty would be the envy of others, which also occurred as predicted. How these things came to pass remained a mystery.

At the time of this writing, eleven years have passed. This client still contacts me occasionally to inform me of his progress and good health. He is happily married, though not to the woman he met after talking to Brandi. The new business that was begun after meeting Brandi lasted only a year before becoming insolvent. However, he loves his current job as a professor and does not believe he has ever felt as happy and fulfilled. My point is that Brandi did not foresee his future, but she was instrumental in enabling its construction. This crucial distinction was famously stated by Antoine de Saint-Exupèry (1950, 152), who wrote, "Your task is not to foresee the future, but to enable it."

6.4 Virtual Boundaries and Interactive Predictions

Can there be such a thing as an interactive prediction in which the target of the prediction helps produce evidence that the prediction will be realized? Certainly! This reminds me of an action taken by William B. Travis (1809–1836) during his historic battle against the Mexican general Antonio López de Santa Anna (1794–1876) at the Alamo in Texas. Because Travis's forces were so badly outnumbered and outgunned, defeat was inevitable. While evacuating the women and children, Travis drew a line in the sand with his sword. He beckoned any soldier who was willing to give his life in defense of the Alamo to step across the line. The rest were asked to leave. His prediction was implied—if you cross the line, you will die fighting for this cause. During the thirteen-day siege, not a single soldier deserted his post or surrendered. As predicted, they all fought to the death.

A familiar concept that helps make sense of this outcome is commitment. By crossing the line in the sand (what researchers refer to as a *virtual boundary*), these individuals made a public commitment. After observing the meaning of their actions, they become more entangled in a prediction that has not been consciously deliberated. While discussing this social dynamic, Milton Erickson (1966) shared the following example,

> Before the patient goes in for that dangerous medical procedure, you ask her if she would be willing to send you the recipe for son-of-a-gun stew once she gets home. And you can explain how much you love son-of-a-gun stew.

When this person agrees to Erickson's request (a virtual boundary), she commits herself to recovery, as implied by the timing of the request (after returning home from the hospital). All of this is achieved without any conscious consideration of what has been predicted (you will quickly recover from surgery).

Rather than viewing hypnosis as a means of exerting special power over others, Erickson treated it more as an experiential device—something that created a virtual boundary, and crossing it committed the person to further action on his or her behalf. Consider the stacking of predictions and virtual boundaries in the following statement, "As soon as you close your eyes and relax into trance, I will use hypnosis to remove the desire to smoke."

A hypnotic protocol is not needed to achieve unconscious goal-oriented engagement. As John Bargh (1992) explains, for priming to work, all that is needed is for words or pictures to be presented in an offhand and unobtrusive manner so that the person does not become aware of the potential influence of the goal-related stimuli. In a clinical setting, whether we are using distraction techniques, trance with dissociated states of consciousness, flow states of consciousness, or the Eastern tradition of wu wei (Chinese for "non-doing"), it all amounts to the same thing—*the surrender of conscious control.*

For example, I said to one client,

> If you are honest with me and yourself about your reasons for wanting to quit smoking, and if we spend some time talking about your history of overcoming extraordinary hardship, you will make up your mind to quit and never look back [implied automaticity].

He then spent the next twenty minutes telling me why he wanted to quit this "filthy" habit.

In this statement, the challenge to be honest was the virtual boundary—an invisible line in the sand. This was a person who *never* backed down from a challenge. Other predictions were also based on aspects of this man's character. He had bragged about being a marine who had worked with special forces, so my offhand comment "never look back" related to a soldier's willingness to die for a cause. Three days later he quit smoking. It was the end of a thirty-year habit.

This is the type of outcome we would expect based on the research. As explained by Peter Gollwitzer (1999), by crossing a virtual boundary a person enters into an implementation mindset (rather than a deliberation mindset), which is characterized by increased action initiation, increased task persistence, and increased optimism in general. This virtual boundary can be anything that demarcates a task, setting, or system and has enough structure to at least imply, if not overtly predict, some outcome.

For clinical applications I sometimes use a chair as a virtual boundary. For example,

> You are not looking at things from your wife's perspective. You need a little more empathy. If you will move over here to this other chair and role play your wife talking to me, you will develop much stronger feelings of empathy.

Obviously, the roleplay will be part of the emotional effect, but there is also a virtual boundary and my confident prediction, which helps formulate unconscious attitudes. Accordingly, Lee and Ariely (2006) found that people's mindsets can change as a function of physical location.

As you will notice in each of these examples, these predictions are stated as an inevitability, which helps produce self-generated images of the future—automatically. Especially once a virtual boundary is crossed, the individual is not likely to become involved with effortful, conscious goal-oriented processing. In contrast, when we stop to establish goals and discuss how they will be achieved, unconscious processing is temporarily sidelined.

6.5 Using Predictions to Answer Unasked Questions

So, does the use of prediction truly qualify as process work? Regarding *conscious* process work, I would argue no. It does not seem to achieve that end.

But *unconscious* process work is a different dynamic. It operates in the dark, quietly producing automatic behaviors that also escape conscious detection. During therapy the therapist does not stop to explain the reasons for using prediction and the anticipated outcomes. It is no longer unconscious process work if the therapist stops to explain the primes or asks the person to deliberate on their effect.

A prediction is an unobtrusive prime that does not trigger conscious involvement (we do not reflect on how the outcomes will be achieved). Instead, prediction activates unconscious processes, such as emotion, cognition, working memory, evaluation, and goal formation. This is all achieved without prescribing a specific means to achieve the end.

For a psychotherapeutic maneuver to qualify as *unconscious* process work, it must address needs (or answer questions) that have yet to be represented (codified) in conscious awareness. A skillful therapist uses prediction as a means of answering emotional questions that are not put to words.

When a client sits for a psychic, they expect direct answers to big questions. For example, "Do you see marriage in my future?" This explicit question has numerous subtextual questions, such as, "Am I someone who others would wish to marry?"

When a client meets with a psychotherapist, the same thing is asked in a different way. For example, "I've never really discussed marriage with anyone I date. Do you think there is anything wrong with me?" But the subtext remains the same—am I someone who others would wish to marry?

The prediction I would offer for such a question might be, "You seem to be saving yourself for just the right person. When you meet him, he will really appreciate the fact that you have not married and divorced your way to him." A little later, I can randomly mention the saying "Good things come to those that wait," which will act as a prime that further reinforces the client's implicit attitudes towards herself by strengthening positive response expectancies.

Something we can see in the last example is that predictions function as a form of validation. People need an external source of authority to confirm internal realities. We construct self-knowledge by asking questions such as, "Am I worthy?" or "Am I capable?" or "Am I loved?" As stated in the *relational self model*, we come to know ourselves through others. As strange as this sounds, we also come to know our potential future through others (due in part to their use of prediction).

Emotional impact is important for gaining the attention of unconscious resources. For that reason, I try to deliver my predictions in an unexpected and emotionally compelling way (hot cognition). It is only after the person engages in skeptical reasoning and asks how I can be so certain of my prediction that I supply her with the probabilistic reasoning behind my claim (cold cognition). Thus, I do not attempt to trick a client into believing that I can read minds or see into the future.

Although I do not know the statistics on every issue that presents in therapy, I keep myself informed of the frequency of certain behaviors given certain circumstances (when X, then Y). This approach dates back to 1954 when Paul Meehl published a revolutionary book, *Clinical Versus Statistical Prediction.*

Clinical prediction refers to the attempt of an expert, such as a clinician, to accurately predict an event. In contrast, statistical predictions are derived from base rates and algorithms. What has been discovered, many times over, is that a good formula frequently matches or outperforms an intuitive clinical prediction. So, whenever possible, I rely on statistical probability.

For example, if I tell a client, "You are going to respond well to therapy, probably with less than ten visits," I know that this is not a baseless prediction. Clinical comparison studies have shown that the average person who engages in psychotherapy is better off by the end of treatment than 80% of those who do not receive treatment (Shapiro and Shapiro, 1982; Smith and Glass, 1977). The average length of treatment in my practice is a dozen visits, and most of the clients provide positive follow-up information.

Often I tell my grieving clients, "As painful as your grief is now, it will start to subside. By one year you will return to normal functioning. After two years, the pain will no longer be noticeable." This prediction is based not only on my professional experience with other grieving clients, but also on various studies.

For example, when looking at grief caused by the death of a pet, results indicate that initially 85.7% of owners experienced at least one symptom of grief, but the occurrence decreased to 35.1% at six months and to 22.4% at one year (Wrobel and Dye, 2003). It hurts to lose a pet! For some, it is like the death of a child.

It hurts equally as bad to have a trusted partner engage in a sexual affair. This loss of trust also requires a prolonged recovery period. So, when the offending partner asks me how long he needs to keep saying he is sorry, I predict a period of about two years if the marriage survives.

If a client says to me, "How long will it take me to get over this relationship? Even though I'm the one that broke up, I can't stop thinking about him and wondering if I made a mistake." My prediction is, "You *may* need a full year. But most likely, you will be dating someone else six months from now." Given the finding that 93% of women become involved in new relationships seven months post-breakup (with a range of 0–13 months), this is a reasonable prediction (Brumbaugh et al., 2015).

And finally, if a client asks, "Will I ever get over this trauma?", I am prepared with a prediction grounded in probability. For those with complex trauma who have been in and out of treatment for many years, my prediction is stated this way, "Major events from your past will always be major events. There is no way I can erase them from your mind. However, if we are patient and persevere with the therapy, you will see some important improvements." In line with this prediction, Morina and colleagues (2014) found that the recovery rate for those with complex trauma and a long history of treatment is 8%. So, a responsible prediction will be modest.

In 2003, I made this modest prediction for a client who fit this category of PTSD clientele (dissociative, suicidal, self-mutilating, alcohol dependent). As often occurs, during her first visit she hinted at what type of progress she was ready to achieve. While making small talk she jokingly stated, "I decided to come back to therapy because I'm too old to be drinking like a teenager." When intoxicated she would become dangerously suicidal. For this client I confidently predicted that therapy would eliminate the drinking problem. This was a safe bet because she was already (unconsciously) implementing a solution to this problem. Her drinking permanently ended after six weeks of therapy.

During the subsequent sixteen years of therapy, she made many other important improvements. At the time of this writing, it has been twelve months since she confidently told me that she no longer needs therapy. She now manages life's daily challenges very well and is pleased and proud of her progress.

If a person who was recently traumatized and immediately sought help asks a prognostic question, my reply is different. I would say,

> It is normal to feel this disturbed after this type of ordeal. But a year from now, you will feel completely different. You may have greater levels of happiness or a stronger sense of purpose and meaning in life. Certainly, you will feel stronger and more resilient.

The recovery rate for those who seek help right after experiencing a single trauma is 89% (Morina et al., 2014). According to Jonathan Haidt (2006) most of these individuals report higher levels of happiness or meaning after twelve months.

When asking yourself "Do I have the right to make such and such prediction," it would be helpful to conceptualize prediction as a vital element in unconscious goal-oriented thinking with prolonged support from unconscious working memory. A therapeutic prediction can maintain implicit attention for years or decades because it addresses unmet needs and deeply experienced desires. Like tipping the first domino, prediction initiates a cascading set of unconscious processes that can lead to new automatic behaviors. You simply cannot go wrong when guiding someone in a positive direction.

Chapter 6 Key Points

- For problems that exceed the capability of conscious intention, credible predictions help activate unconscious goal-oriented problem solving, which includes implicit experiential knowledge and persistence despite setbacks.

- Predictions should be framed loosely within time and space, typically aiming at a remote future.
- Process-oriented predictions are ambiguous, pointing to what can happen while avoiding a discussion of how it will happen.
- Interactive predictions employ *if/then* contingencies (*if* you do X, *then* Y will occur).
- Use predictions that are emotionally compelling but also responsible and probable.
- Trust your implicit perceptions and intuitive knowledge. If you do not feel comfortable with a certain prediction, then do not make it.

References

Bargh, John A. 1992. "The Ecology of Automaticity: Toward Establishing the Conditions Needed to Produce Automatic Processing Effects." *The American Journal of Psychology* 105 (2): 181–199. doi:10.2307/1423027.

Brumbaugh, Claudia C., and R. Chris Fraley. 2015. "Too Fast, Too Soon?: An Empirical Investigation into Rebound Relationships." *Journal of Social and Personal Relationships* 32 (1): 99–118. doi:10.1177/0265407514525086.

Erickson, Milton H. 1966. *A Lecture by Milton H. Erickson, Houston, February 18, 1966.* (Audio Recording No. CD/EMH.66.2.18). Phoenix, AZ: The Milton H. Erickson Foundation Archives.

Erickson, Milton H., and Sidney Rosen. 1982. *My Voice Will Go with You: The Teaching Tales of Milton H. Erickson, M.D.* New York: W. W. Norton & Company.

Erickson, Milton H., and Ernest L. Rossi. 1975. "Varieties of Double Bind." In *The Collected Works of Milton H. Erickson, Volume 2, Basic Hypnotic Induction & Suggestion*, 161–180. Phoenix, AZ: Milton H. Erickson Foundation.

Gilovich, Thomas, Margaret Kerr, and Victoria H. Medvec. 1993. "Effect of Temporal Perspective on Subjective Confidence." *Journal of Personality and Social Psychology* 64 (4): 552–560. doi:10.1037/0022-3514.64.4.552.

Gollwitzer, Peter M. 1999. "Deliberative versus Implemental Mindsets in the Control of Action." In *Dual-Process Theories in Social Psychology*, edited by Shelly Chaiken and Yaacov Trope, 403–422. New York: Guilford Press.

Haidt, Jonathan. 2006. *The Happiness Hypothesis: Finding Modern Truth in Ancient Wisdom.* New York: Basic Books.

Kirsch, Irving. 1990. *Changing Expectations: A Key to Effective Psychotherapy*. Belmont, CA: Thomson Brooks/Cole Publishing.

Kirsch, Irving, Guy Montgomery, and Guy Sapirstein. 1995. "Hypnosis as an Adjunct to Cognitive-Behavioral Psychotherapy: A Meta-Analysis." *Journal of Consulting and Clinical Psychology* 63 (2): 214–220. doi:10.1037/0022-006X.63.2.214.

Lee, Leonard, and Dan Ariely. 2006. "Shopping Goals, Goal Concreteness, and Conditional Promotions." *Journal of Consumer Research* 33 (1): 60–70. doi:10.1086/504136.

Meehl, Paul E. 1954. *Clinical Versus Statistical Prediction: A Theoretical Analysis and a Review of the Evidence.* Brattleboro, VT: Echo Point Books & Media.

Miller, Scott D. 2017. "The Missing Link: Why 80% of People Who Could Benefit Will Never See a Therapist." *scottdmiller.com.* https://www.scottdmiller.com/the-missing-link-why-80-of-people-who-could-benefit-will-never-see-a-therapist.

Miller, Scott D., and Mark Hubble. 2017. "How Psychotherapy Lost Its Magick: The Art of Healing in an Age of Science." *Psychotherapy Networker*, 2017. https://www.psychotherapynetworker.org/magazine/article/1077/how-psychotherapy-lost-its-magick.

Morina, Nexhmedin, Jelte M. Wicherts, Jakob Lobbrecht, and Stefan Priebe. 2014. "Remission from Post-Traumatic Stress Disorder in Adults: A Systematic Review and Meta-Analysis of Long Term Outcome Studies." *Clinical Psychology Review* 34 (3): 249–255. doi:10.1016/j.cpr.2014.03.002.

Popper, Karl. 1977. *Unended Quest*. New York: Routledge.

Saint-Exupéry, Antoine de. 1950. *The Wisdom of the Sands*. Translated by S. Gilbert. New York:Harcourt, Brace and Company.

Shapiro, David A., and Diana Shapiro. 1982. "Meta-Analysis of Comparative Therapy Outcome Studies: A Replication and Refinement." *Psychological Bulletin* 92 (3): 581–604. doi:10.1037/0033-2909.92.3.581.

Smith, Mary L., and Gene V. Glass. 1977. "Meta-Analysis of Psychotherapy Outcome Studies." *American Psychologist* 32 (9): 752–760. doi:10.1037/0003-066X.32.9.752.

Surbled, Georges. "Hypnotism." In *Catholic Encyclopedia*, Vol. 7, 604–610. New York: Encyclopedia Press. https://en.wikisource.org/wiki/Catholic_Encyclopedia_(1913)/Hypnotism.

Trope, Yaacov, and Nira Liberman. 2010. "Construal-Level Theory of Psychological Distance." *Psychological Review* 117 (2): 440–463. doi:10.1037/a0018963.

Wrobel, Thomas A., and Amanda L. Dye. 2003. "Grieving Pet Death: Normative, Gender, and Attachment Issues." *OMEGA – Journal of Death and Dying* 47 (4): 385–393. doi:10.2190/QYV5-LLJ1-T043-U0F9.

7 Reimagining

In *Man's Search for Meaning*, Viktor Frankl (1946) describes his therapeutic approach to a situation in which circumstance seems to dictate fate. Frankl's patient was an elderly physician in a state of severe depression. He was struggling with the loss of his wife, who had died two years previous. The lonely widower told Frankl, "I loved her above all else."

Frankl responded by asking the grieving widower, "What would have happened, Doctor, if you had died first, and your wife would have had to survive you?" The patient responded with deep emotionality, "Oh, for her this would have been terrible; how she would have suffered!"

Frankl replied, "You see, Doctor, such suffering has been spared her, and it was you who have spared her this suffering—to be sure, at the price that now you have to survive and mourn her."

After hearing this statement, the man did not say anything else. He just shook Frankl's hand and calmly left the office.

Frankl's interpretation of these events was that suffering ceases to be suffering the moment it finds a meaning, such as the meaning of a sacrifice. Dissecting his technique, we can see that Frankl used a special type of question to alter the meaning of his patient's past. Whenever someone is asked "*What if* such and such had happened?", attention automatically shifts to the past, but not the actual past. It is a reimagined past in which alterative realities are speculated upon during an unconscious evaluative process.

While discussing the significance of personal narratives, Donald Meichenbaum (2014) argued that certain questions have greater therapeutic value than others. As a rule, he avoids questions that start with *why* (which engages critical conscious analysis) and instead uses questions starting with *what* or *how*. As we see in Frankl's case example, when *what* is followed by *if*, or *how* is followed by *could*, an automatic process of reimagining is prompted.

Certainly, Frankl's intervention would have fallen flat if the man had not spontaneously reimagined his wife alone and heartbroken. This evaluative process can occur instantaneously since it draws on the extraordinary speed of unconscious processing.

In order to enrich our clinical perspective with scientifically tested ideas, it is useful to consider new discoveries coming from temporal self-appraisal theory

DOI: 10.4324/9781003127208-7

(TSA). The essential finding from this line of research is that individuals' sense of self is highly dependent on the perspective from which they view their past. This is relevant to reimagining because this technique is meant to change people's perceptions of themselves in both the past and the future.

Using experimental manipulations, TSA researchers have shown that the more distant a past self becomes, the less of an impact it has on the current self. In the clinical setting, the most extreme version of this self-protective distancing would be repression (dissociative amnesia), such that a past self is entirely forgotten. This would explain why, after repressed memories unexpectedly burst into conscious awareness, severe emotional problems often emerge.

Research has also shown that any modification to a past construction of self will change the feelings and behaviors of a current self. For example, it was found that people feel better about their current selves when induced to feel close to past achievements (Peetz and Wilson, 2008). This increase in proximity is achieved by processing these events more frequently, describing them more vividly, or using concrete images to represent them. Questions that point to a past glory include "*What* was your proudest moment?", "*Who* did you discuss this with?", and "*How* did you find the courage to do that?"

Accordingly, the feeling of distance from former *shortcomings* also helps improve self-perception. Objects or events are made more distal by using questions such as "How long ago was that?", "Could that ever happen here?", or "How have you changed since then?" Distance is also achieved by using abstract words to describe the basic gist of things and avoiding sensory details (Wilson and Ross, 2003).

These discoveries are relevant to the therapeutic endeavor, but there is no reason to expect a temporary change in self-perception to produce lasting change. To achieve this, it is necessary to create momentum—there must be some intellectual process work (e.g., new goals, new beliefs, new attitudes) that carries forward beyond the external support provided by the therapist. When the process work is unconscious, its impact is extended beyond the small, flickering spotlight of conscious awareness.

7.1 Priming Downward Counterfactuals

Returning to Frankl's case, we can see that his question served as a prime. From there, the creative capacity of unconscious imagination took over. This imagined reality (his wife outliving him) was of course fictional. Using scientific terminology, we would call this *downward counterfactual thinking* (reimagining the past as something that could have been worse). Researchers call it *upward counterfactuals* when reimagining the past as something that could have been much better.

Undoubtedly, the man had come to Frankl with his emotional and cognitive systems fixated on how the past could have been better—if only she hadn't died, if only I had done more to help her! As shown by Sanna (2000), upward counterfactuals (reimagining a better past) tend to increase negative feelings, such as regret, remorse, and disappointment. In contrast, downward counterfactuals compare the recollected outcome to worse possible outcomes. This tends to increase positive feelings, such as joy, satisfaction, and relief. In this example, Frankl's use of reimagining is so subtle and eloquent that it almost escapes detection. There are also hidden benefits that we would not see without considering the research.

A study by Galinsky and Moskowitz's (2000) showed that when primed to engaged in counterfactual thinking (reimagining), people will problem solve more effectively. In laboratory tests, the effect is dramatic, with a 56% rate of improvement relative to those in the no-prime control condition. The increase in success seems to come from an increased ability to consider alternatives while avoiding old, ineffective solutions (mental sets). This discovery is important for care providers because one of the essential tasks in therapy is to stimulate clients to move beyond old, ineffective solutions. In other words, reimagining not only helps people progress emotionally but also increases their effectiveness at problem solving.

7.2 Generating Alternative Representations

Imagine, *what if* psychotherapists had the ability to edit problematic life experiences just as medical doctors are starting to use gene editing to alter DNA and either delete sections or replace them with alternate adaptive sequences. By changing a person's past, we theoretically change the blueprints for the constitution of the psyche. According to a globally respected researcher in trauma, Chris Brewin (2018), psychological editing techniques, such as *imagery rescripting* and viewing the scene from other perspectives (reimagining), enable therapists to generate alternative representations that are particularly effective at competing with and inhibiting problematic memories. As argued in the study of epigenetics, when we change the psyche, we change the traces of traumatic events that became encoded in DNA (Jiang et al., 2019).

Before looking at the history and science of reimagining, I would like to illustrate its use. In this case, I was teaching an audience of mental health professionals about the benefits of changing the past to create a new future. Fortunately, I was able to demonstrate the technique with a woman from the audience.

Her complaint was that she had lived her entire life caught in a pattern of self-destructive behavior. As she stated, "Many times in my life I find that I have put myself in violent situations … It makes no sense … It is as if that is the way that I will survive."

The precipitating event, which she continued to have strong feelings about, was her birth. She said this experience was violent, and she had been taken from her mother for an immediate blood transfusion. Her intellectual understanding of the event indicated that she had discussed it with her parents.

I explained to her that while reimagining her past, I would help her keep the essential parts of her memory intact (the same basic story), which in this case was the fact that she was born with a blood incompatibility problem and required emergency care. I told her that just some of the minor details would be changed. As with most clients plagued by disturbing memories, she was eager to have the traumatic memory altered.

When using this technique, I do not attempt to alter any details until the story reaches its apex—the moment at which the situation becomes unbearable. For her, it was the moment the nurse tore her away from her mother.

While she was narrating this story, I collected sensory details using a first-person perspective in present tense, "What do you see? … Who is holding you? … How does it feel?" The tone of her voice and emotion on her face made it clear that she was reliving the traumatic event. Wincing, she exclaimed that something was stuck into her heel, that she was in pain, and that everyone was panicking.

Next, I asked what would make her feel better. As with most people caught in a traumatic experience, she could not say what she needed. I asked, "Would it help if I could get your mother to you?" She cried out as a frightened child, "Yes!" So, I suggested that her mother had rushed to her and was holding her in her arms. I said that she was looking into her mother's eyes as her mother comforted her with words of love. I suggested that her mother's comfort made the hurt and fear vanish.

While fully absorbing her in all the sensory details of a mother-infant attachment experience, I told her that she had a right to be in her mother's arms, and she could stay there as long as she would like.

Having reimagined her past, I then took her far into her future, beyond the moment of her mother's death as an elderly woman. Mirroring the new memories created for her birth, I assured her that she would still be able to feel her mother's arms around her, feel her love, and hear her words of wisdom whenever she needed them, even from beyond the grave.

A few months later, I was involved in a case discussion during which other professionals watched a video of this demonstration and offered their critiques. It was an international webinar involving institutes from around the world. A woman sitting in the front row of the French institute was particularly vocal about the positive aspects of the therapy, while others from the United States disagreed and stated concerns about the risks of implanting false memories.

During this dispute, I remained silent. As the woman in France tried to make the point that this technique is empowering and promotes personal choice, she was forcefully challenged by the skeptics, who asked how she could be so certain that things had turned out well for this demonstration subject. Her response was, "I KNOW because I am that woman!"

Though we had all just watched a video of my work with her, she was only recognized by her French colleagues and myself. The person sitting next to me exclaimed, "My God! She has lost over twenty pounds! She doesn't look like the same person." More than the weight loss, I was pleased to see the new strength that emanated from her. She was no longer apologetic and hiding behind others. She spoke as someone who knew that she had a right to exist and to claim her spot within the world.

My hope is that the reader will recognize that the act of reimagining the past parallels any *as if* process. It is an appeal to the client's unconscious intelligence, creative capacity, and right to experience choice. As we can see from a long history of clinical practice and recent research, the exercise in reimagining is not frivolous. Similar to the notion of epigenetics changing DNA, we can say that by editing the most toxic experiences from this woman's autobiographical narrative and replacing them with more adaptive experiences, her psychological self was reconstituted—with modifications to attitudes, beliefs, and expectations processed outside of conscious awareness. The significance of such an exercise can hardly be understated. I think Donald Meichenbaum (2014, 20) put it well when he said, "Bad things happen to a lot of people. Future wellbeing depends more so on the stories people create as a result of what has occurred, what conclusions they draw about themselves and others, and about the future."

To the best of my knowledge, Pierre Janet (1859–1947) was the first to describe this powerful technique in his paper titled "Histoire d'une idée fixe" (Janet, 1894). His methodology was illustrated with the case of Marie, who Janet cured of psychogenic blindness after using "imagery replacement."

The problem had begun when Marie was forced to share a bed with a child whose face was disfigured by impetigo (a highly contagious skin infection). That night, Marie had stared at the child's face in terror, fearing that she would suffer the same fate. Janet used hypnosis to help her relive the event but imagine that the child's face was normal.

To increase proximity to these new positive memories, Janet added other sensory details, such as Marie stroking the girl's hair and face, and Marie feeling pleased that the girl was so friendly. Janet reports that after she accepted the new memory, her symptoms disappeared.

In another example of imagery replacement, Janet reported the case of Justine, who developed a morbid fear of death after helping her mother—a nurse—treat dying patients. Traumatized by the experience, Justine became haunted by intrusive images of naked corpses, including a Chinese general that she had seen. While experiencing flashbacks, Justine would be thrown into hysterical seizures. Using hypnosis, Janet had her produce a comic image of the general dancing. Following this, Justine became symptom free (Lynn et al., 2012). As will be further discussed in section 7.4, the chronic overactivation of the adolescent's fear was counter-regulated through the addition of humor.

Thus, one of Janet's most important technical contributions to the therapeutic endeavor is the clinical application of memory reconsolidation, in which mental representations held in long-term memory are destabilized by being brought into the conscious field. In this destabilized state, parts of the memory are modified or enhanced, resulting in a reorganization of attitudes and emotions. The reorganized memory is then reconsolidated and returned to long-term storage, where it serves as a foundation for unconscious processing.

This same method continues to be practiced in a variety of modalities. Within the hypnotherapeutic context, Milton Erickson provided a detailed account of his use of strategic memory reconsolidation to help a woman access and reimagine traumatic memories from childhood (Erickson and Rossi, 1989). In this case, Erickson introduced a kind elderly gentleman, known as the February Man, who comes to the woman's aid during some of her most difficult moments in childhood. In this context, suggestions for age regression and altered states of consciousness helped increase the emotional saliency of the therapeutic experience.

Working in a group therapy setting, Bob and Mary Goulding (1979) describe the same methodology but without eliciting a trance state. Rather than using the concept of age regression, clients are taught to access a *child ego state* and then recall difficult moments in childhood. The aim of redecision therapy (RT) is to help clients accept responsibility for moving from a victim position to one of personal empowerment. This is achieved by having group members creatively reimagine early scenes in their childhoods in a way that improves upon early decisions about self and others.

Within the context of CBT, *imagery rescripting* (IR) has been introduced as a means to change emotional memories (Smucker et al., 1995). In IR therapy, disturbing mental images are modified in order to reduce associated negative emotions and pathological schemas associated with the traumatic event(s). The use of guided imagery is described as a form of exposure therapy that is supplemented with cognitive restructuring. The introduction of "mastery imagery" is used to create more adaptive schemas versus traumatic representations of vulnerability, isolation, powerlessness, anger, betrayal, etc. An interesting component of this work is that clients are asked to write out the reimagined scenario, thus increasing the probability of memory change. There is now a great deal of outcome research supporting this methodology for reducing PTSD symptomatology (e.g., Arntz, 2012).

Lastly, the Freudian analyst Jacques Lacan (1901–1981) argued that process work is by necessity imaginative and should lead to the symbolic rewriting of history. In contrast to the approach described in this chapter, Lacan did not believe that the therapist can explain to the client that the past needs to be reimagined. He assumed this would elicit aggression. Lacan viewed his therapy as paradoxical, "the praxis of analysis is obliged to advance toward a conquest of the truth via the pathways of deception" (Lacan and Mehlman, 1987, 95).

What Lacan overlooked was the enthusiasm and childlike joy that clients experience when they are given permission to "play with the past." If we think of consciousness as being something like a canvas, then it is easy to understand why any validation of a person's creative expression upon that canvas brings joy—not anger. It is the same as when you admire someone's artwork (child or adult) and affirm the beauty you see in their creation.

The first question some people ask about reimagining the past is whether this might produce false memories. The answer is almost certainly that it does. Research has shown that new memories are created *anytime* mental representations held in long-term memory are destabilized by being brought into the conscious field. When working with childhood memories, asking a person to imagine an experience and add some sensory detail is often enough to render the details of the imaginative experience as indistinguishable from the preexisting memory (Garry et al., 1996).

As another example, researchers Loftus and Pickrell (1995) found that by merely having subjects discuss "false" memories alongside "true" memories, they were able to detect obvious revisions in 25% of subjects. Of course, even the "true" memories are likely constructions that have evolved over time. As Coyle (1997) puts it, science suggests that when people recall the past, they make educated guesses about what must have happened. On average, it appears that nearly half of all memory content is confabulated (Scoboria et al., 2017).

Memory is continually reconstructed. Minor details are constantly changing, even for major life events. For memory that is considered continuous, the basic gist of the memory remains the same. Similarly, while the basic gist of what we expect for the future remains unchanged, the details of our future are constantly reimagined.

We identify with our past, so the idea that our memories are malleable can be difficult to accept. Current Western culture is much more comfortable treating our imagined future as malleable. But imaginative constructionism is bidirectional, it goes backwards in time as easily as it goes forward. The human mind is not a video recorder. As shown by researchers, such as Tulving and Craik (2005), memory is essentially a reconstructive process that is significantly impacted by imagination and priming effects, which occur during memory retrieval.

As ominous as this sounds, we should recognize that the real problem is not that memories can be altered. People's expectations for the future can also be altered, and this too can produce therapeutic effects. The greater problem is fatalistic psychotherapies—those that focus on pathologizing the client or alienating the client from important sources of social support.

At the opposite end of the spectrum, competency-oriented psychotherapies nurture a growth-oriented mindset focused on the goodness of one's mind and body as well as one's past and future experiences. Therapies that produce the most positive outcomes also place a strong emphasis on alliance building (inside and outside the consultation room) and relationship repair.

Regarding memory, ethical therapy utilizes any continuous memory construction as a stabilizing force in the psyche. In contrast, unethical therapy takes productive, integrated memories and transforms them into something toxic and destructive (e.g., "maybe you were sexually abused and just don't remember it"). While there is impressive research indicating that repressed memories (dissociative amnesia) do exist, it is arguably unethical to engage in "memory recovery work." The risk of inducing iatrogenic trauma is too great. Furthermore, there has never been a credible body of evidence indicating that memory recovery produces therapeutic benefit.

As Freud's insight therapy began to dominate the field, Morton Prince (1912, 420) attempted to make clear the limitations of memory recovery, "The awakening of dormant memories of past experiences is mainly of importance for the purpose of giving us exact information of *what* we need to modify, not necessarily for the purpose of effecting the modification."

In other words, the realization of what is bothering you does not change the psychological impact of these mental representations. Even after achieving insight, innumerable memories, attitudes, emotions, and motivations remain linked to the event as interactive components operating outside of conscious awareness. As argued by Erickson, for meaningful change to follow, a creative reorganization of these mental representations must occur at an unconscious level (Erickson and Rossi, 1979).

In one of the earliest attempts to conceptually model how this type of reorganization is achieved, Morton Prince (1912, 416) distinguished two types of memory reconstruction:

1. "A new setting with strong affects may be artificially created so that the perception acquires another equally strong meaning and intent."
2. "[B]ring into consciousness the setting and the past experiences … and reform it by introducing new elements, including new emotions and feelings."

In the first technique, Prince is talking about alterations to semantic memory (the meaning of past events). This is often referred to in clinical literature as reframing. In the second, Prince is referring to alterations to episodic memory (the content and sequence of past events). Thus, when working with the past, we have two clinical options—either change the meaning of a past event or change the memory of what occurred. However, when considering the therapeutic benefits of reimagining, it is not just the past that we should be interested in.

7.3 Priming Upward Prefactuals

As William James (1890) phrased it, we live in the "specious present," which means our perceptions of *what is* are superficially plausible, but inaccurate. James goes on to explain, "the knowledge of some other part of the stream [of consciousness], past or future, near or remote, is always mixed in with our knowledge of the present thing" (1890, vol. I, 1405). Transference relationships would be a classic example of the past shaping our understanding of the present. And, self-fulfilling prophecy is an example of an anticipated future defining our understanding of the present.

For example, when the phone rings, is that good or bad? Should you run to the phone or block that caller? This all depends on the future, as constructed through imagination and enriched by stories about the past.

This is why religion (which seeks to define the very beginning of existence and the ultimate end) has such a close relationship to meaning. If you control the final chapter of the autobiographical narrative (i.e., this will take you to heaven or hell), then you control the meaning of everything else that comes before. This is not to discount the importance of institutions that make predictions and produce narratives (science being one of them), but rather to highlight the role of imagination in defining reality.

Returning to the research, in TSA we see evidence of a bidirectional link between *memory* and *future expectations*. As argued by Ross and Wilson (2001), we carry constructions of past and future selves, each able to influence the other. These self-referential relationships are interdependent, which means you cannot change one without changing the other.

Turning to research on memory and expectation, the emerging consensus within the scientific community is that the ability to simulate personal future events relies heavily on the ability to remember a continuous past (memory integration). Thus, the relationship between these two dimensions of temporal reality is circular rather than linear.

What has been shown is that processes, such as motivation, attitudes, decisions, and behavior, can be affected by speculation on what the future might be even though these future selves are always hypothetical or imagined. What this means for clinical work is that a damaged sense of self can be repaired by going back into the past or forward into the future.

Thus, psychotherapists should be prepared to work in all three dimensions of temporal reality. Or, as Erickson said to a patient in preparation for unconscious process work, "You can find yourself ranging into the past, the present, or the future as your unconscious selects the most appropriate means of dealing with that" (Erickson and Rossi, 1979, 26).

Before beginning a discussion of the therapeutic application of prefactual thinking (which simply means to think hypothetically and imaginatively about the future), I will demonstrate its therapeutic application with a case example. This was a life-and-death situation that required more technical versatility than I was accustomed to using.

The client was a 35-year-old male who had endured an extremely abusive childhood. His mother had been a heroin addict who sometimes smashed his head up against the post of his bunkbed when she could not find a fix for her drug habit. On more than one occasion, he found her unconscious with a needle still in her arm. When he turned 14, his mother kicked him out of the house. With no place to go, he joined a violent street gang. Shortly after, he became addicted to crystal methamphetamine (meth). This drug had ruled his life for almost two decades. Now he was in my office in a very bad condition.

With bloodshot eyes and his body shaking, he said to me, "I'm ready to blow my f-cking brains out!" The danger was imminent. He had the gun in his car.

Four years prior, he had placed a gun in his mouth and pulled the trigger, but he turned his head at the last minute so the bullet went into the wall. His neighbors called the police. He was charged with unlawful discharge of a weapon, which is a felony charge. This resulted in lots of legal fees, the loss of his job, and him becoming unemployable. The mother of his son had tried for years to support him. But his actions had become too threatening, so she obtained a restraining order and told him that he was no longer welcome in the home. To make matters worse, with no place to sleep and no money for drugs, he was in a state of acute withdrawal.

He informed me that I was probably the last person he would be speaking to. I hoped that because he had gone to the trouble to come in for therapy he secretly wanted to live. This man was reaching out for help, and I was the person he had chosen during his darkest hour.

I knew better than to bring up his past, because it would further destabilize him. So, I decided to use hypnosis to try and help his body relax and to communicate some degree of hope. After getting him to agree to close his eyes, I used a hypnotic context to deliver a series of primes: images of him seeing his son graduate in the future, his body in a relaxed and comfortable state, etc. The problem was that, at that moment, he hated everyone and everything, including his body and his failed efforts as a father.

After opening his eyes and with his arms and legs tremoring violently, the man sarcastically declared, "Thanks a lot Doc. Before coming to see you, I thought I might kill myself. Now I f-cking know I'm going to do it!" He glanced over his shoulder towards his car—the location of the gun. Feeling intense pressure, I decided that I needed to act quickly and with a more effective approach.

I admitted my failure and asked him for another chance. This time I did not say anything about relaxation or future happiness. Instead, I said,

> Okay, I know you can close your eyes. [I wait for him to comply] Now, nod if you can imagine seeing your son standing outside my office—behind the building and out of sight. [He nods] Good! Now imagine a man slowly approaching. [My voice becomes deep and ominous] Someone who has bad intent. Someone who is a PREDATOR and a PERVERT! [Long silence] Now your 12-year-old son is standing out there all alone. And this predator is getting ready to tell your son to drop his pants. Do you want to be dead in the grave? [Long silence] Or, do you want to still be around so that you can do something about this situation? [I see his jaw and fists clench] Okay good! Step in between this man and your son. Tell your son that he can come inside my office so that he does not see what happens next. I promise, I will keep him safe in here with me. [Long silence] Now you are free to do with this person as you wish. It doesn't matter what you do. Just make certain he is in no position to ever threaten your son again.

My client spent a while with this imagery, which was essentially an internal set of self-expanding primes. The story took on a life of its own and did not require my continued narration.

Ironically, after opening his eyes his body was visibly relaxed. His arms and legs were still. When I asked what he had done to the predator, with a very serious expression he told me that I didn't want to know.

He then confessed to me that he needed help getting off this "damn drug." He was able to recognize that meth had destroyed his life. Worst of all, it made him unavailable as a father. Following the unconscious process work, his attitudes shifted. Sobriety replaced suicide as his top priority.

With a half-chuckle he said, "No offense to you Doc, but I think I need more help than what you can do for me here in this office." I suggested the Salvation Army, and he agreed. With nowhere else to go, we decided he should drive straight from my office to their drug rehabilitation center. I asked if the gun was in his car. It was. So, I recommended he take it to a friend who would keep it for him while he was working on his sobriety. I did not think that the Salvation Army would welcome firearms. He agreed.

The visualization of a hypothetical future got him started. The Salvation Army got him sober. And AA gave him the structure, education, and social support he needed to stay sober. His last visit to my office was four years later. At that time, he was enjoying a close relationship with his son and a one-day-at-a-time life of sobriety. Before leaving, he made certain to hand me my own copy of the "Big Book" (the foundational text for Alcoholics Anonymous), for which I was grateful.

If while reading this story some part of you was imagining what to do with a suicidal client and examining various alternatives, then you were engaging in prefactual thinking. This creative capacity occurs automatically and sometimes without conscious attention.

Whenever you envision yourself acting in the future and pursuing a positive alternative, it is known as an *upward prefactual*. If you envision yourself picking an undesirable course of action, it is known as a *downward prefactual*. It is the downward frame that is common amongst severely depressed individuals, such as my client. Whenever he imagined the future, all he could see was him making things worse. By contrast, when I gave him the opportunity to utilize all his aggression and rage for the sake of (hypothetically) saving his son's life, it produced an upward prefactual—the antidote to depression.

7.4 The Counter-regulation of Emotion

If we go beyond the narrow frame of cognitive psychology, which is mostly interested in thoughts, and consider the role of emotion in producing behavior, we find a different purpose for reimagining our past or our future. Before explaining this, I will provide a concrete example.

A woman in her mid-40s came to me for help with depression. She lived alone and got most of her social needs met through work. Therefore, it affected her deeply when she felt that she was being mistreated or taken advantage of at work. While describing her struggles, she explained that she felt unappreciated and disempowered. As she put it, "I do not feel like I have a voice there."

Whenever a client engages in the use of metaphor, you can be certain that there is something there worth exploring. I decided I would use imaginative involvement to initiate unconscious process work.

This process begins by identifying a memory of the past (or image of the future) that is accessible to conscious awareness but not normally considered during day-to-day problem solving. So, I asked her, "When is the first time you remember feeling that you have no voice?" After a brief pause, she said it was her childhood. Her father had been a violent alcoholic who beat her mother. She said that she had many memories of fearing for her mother's survival. I instructed her to go back to one of the earliest memories that she felt able to discuss with me.

In this memory, she was four years old and hiding at the top of the stairwell. It was late at night, and she was supposed to be in bed. She saw her father screaming at her mother and raising his arms in the air ready to strike her. Her mother was screaming. My client said she recalled feeling fearful that he would kill her. She wanted to run down the stairs and help her mother. But her body would not move. She was frozen in terror. She wished to be able to scream out, "Stop it!" But she could not speak.

After hearing her story, I had her close her eyes and imagine that she had returned to this moment. I guided her perception of what was occurring while adding some new elements. In this reimagined version, she found in her hand a magic wand, which was given to her by a fairy princess. With her wand she had the courage to walk down the stairs and approach her father. I suggested that by waving the wand she could freeze her father in place. In this state he would be unable to move and unable to talk. But I assured her that he could hear everything she had to say.

I then prompted my client to give her father the lecture she had always wished to give him but had never been able to. I invited her to tell him what he needed to hear in order to be a better father and husband. The story ended with her unfreezing her father and then supervising his apologies to her mother. With the wand still in hand, she had the assurance that she could refreeze him if he did not behave correctly. This process of creative reimagining lasted approximately twenty minutes.

Whether going into the future (prospective) or the past (retrospective), my primary reason for helping clients reimagine their autobiographical narrative is to provide an opportunity to exercise choice. For a client who has been demoralized by helplessness, failure, boundary violations, abandonment, or rejection, the opportunity to exercise choice is like giving oxygen to an accident victim suffering shock. It seems to be a vital resource in the care of human consciousness.

More specific to this case, my intention was to use creative play to help her find her voice—whatever that meant to her subjective unconscious. It was also an opportunity for her to learn more about the possibility of relationship repair by teaching her father in virtual reality the steps needed to repair his marriage.

Although I did not know it at the time, researchers Driskell, Copper, and Moran (1994) found that the optimal amount of time to devote to mental practice is twenty minutes. More or less time spent in mental simulation has been shown to reduce the benefits. Also, the longer one waits between mental practice and actual performance, the smaller the effect. This is why I encourage clients to use the new skills acquired in therapy at the first available opportunity. For this woman, it meant using her voice at work the next day, which she did.

A week later she returned to my office psychologically transformed. She was no longer depressed and said she had a new perspective on the importance of her role in the office. She now saw that her colleagues appreciated her contributions. It was as if she was looking at her social world through a new lens.

So why did this imaginative involvement in her past make such a big difference? There may be many reasons. Looking to contemporary research, it has been found that acquiring a sense of control over what was happening during a moment of trial increases resilience to adversity. This sense of personal ability (self-efficacy) enables patients to employ inner capacities and experiential learnings to achieve their objectives. As Albert Bandura (2000, 75) puts it, "Unless people believe that they can produce desired effects and forestall undesired ones by their actions, they have little incentive to act." By reimagining her past, this woman was afforded the *feeling* of self-efficacy.

It can also be argued that the fantasy experience helped facilitate an emotional reversal. During her regression to the past, this woman went from being in a frozen state of terror to boldly asserting her wishes with her father (the most powerful figure in her psychological world).

Consider the differences in fear-based thought versus courage-based thought. Consider the changes in physiology. In the mental simulation she went from being paralyzed to freely moving about the house, probably with a straight spine and firmly set jaw. There were other emotions involved as well: hope that her father would behave better in the future, the sheer delight of owning a magical wand, and the pride that came from protecting her mother. In this single act of mental simulation, the utility of all these previously unknown emotions was discovered. With each of these different emotional frames come different sets of options and automatic behaviors. In other words, emotional experiences are closely connected to action tendencies and emotion congruent thoughts. Happy people think happy thoughts and do happy things, whereas angry people think angry thoughts and do angry things.

If you think of each emotional set as a window into possible solutions for a problem, it is not surprising that emotionally fluid individuals are more creative problem solvers. Instead of having only one perspective from which to view the problem, each new emotion becomes a new angle from which the problem is perceived. As for my client, she gained access to a greater variety of emotional states than she had dared use in the past. Consequently, she was no longer trapped in her old *mental set.*

A line of research that helps inform our understanding of these dynamics is the study of *counter-regulation*. Simply put, counter-regulation is an automatic quality of mind in which the affective quality of an initial emotional experience is reversed by the emergence of another competing emotion. This is referred to as *affect neutralization*.

For healthy individuals, emotions come and go rather quickly, lasting an average of only seven minutes before being neutralized. Because strong emotions are beyond intentional control, it is important for individuals to learn how to automatically engage this implicit emotion regulation mechanism, which reduces the intensity and duration of emotional states.

In an important discovery, known as the *counter-regulation principle*, Klaus Rothermund (2011) found that one way this implicit emotion regulation system functions is by automatically moving attention to stimuli that are opposite in valence to the current affective motivational focus.

You can find examples of this in your own personal experience—assuming you are not a severely traumatized individual with rigid emotional sets. For example, think of the last time you were angry at your child, perhaps for disobeying you. As you spoke in angry, stern tones, your thoughts likely went to all the reasons why he or she should have known better. For these few moments the child gets no sympathy from you. But three minutes later you catch a glimpse of your child looking down at the ground. You suddenly realize how small the child feels, and your anger is replaced with compassion and reconciliatory tones. Researchers Schwager and Rothermund (2013) point out the importance of this unconscious mechanism in preventing any one emotion (positive or negative) from growing into an exaggerated state or from developing into chronic states of anger, depression, anxiety, or Pollyannaish optimism.

The therapeutic application for this principle is that during imaginative involvement we can manually guide the client's attention to new situational details so that counter-regulation is enacted. The experience for the client is one of liberation, and the more emotional shifts you help facilitate, the greater the sense of freedom. Especially for those clients who have been trying to avoid feeling anything about a past event, it is very helpful to show how a person can feel many different ways about the same event.

With one severely traumatized client who had been emotionally flat her entire adult life, I had her retell an experience with rape and explain what about it made her feel fearful—an emotional state that would be easily within reach. After supporting and validating that emotional state, I helped her reimagine the event in a way that enabled her to feel angry. We achieved this by having her focus on the face of the aggressor. To increase her sense of personal power, I had her imagine a gun in her hand (her hobby is shooting guns). The next emotion was sadness. Then, I helped her shift to positive emotions. She felt peace while imagining herself looking at her white coverup blowing in the wind. She went on to experience self-compassion and then hope. This was all achieved within a context of safety and freedom of choice. It is not therapeutic to simply relive a traumatic experience. The past must be reimagined in a way that leads to more fluid states of consciousness. By the end of the session, my client was not only more animated and talkative but also much less fearful of her life experiences.

To broaden our emotional perspective, we must be willing to "experiment" with feeling different emotions while reflecting on a singular event. Reimagining something that has already taken place, but with new emotional states, is not only a boost to unconscious problem solving but conscious awareness expands as well. The same hold true when reimagining the future—allowing yourself to experience a variety of outcomes with many different emotional reactions to each.

Careful problem solvers are good at counter-regulation. They seek to experience their world with as many emotional perspectives as possible. Each new feeling state provides its own specialized systems of logic and behavioral patterns. Like any other skill, the capacity to intentionally switch between feeling states increases with practice and while engaging in creative reimagining, which is essential to experiencing choice.

7.5 Choice Is Not the Same as Free Will

The Russian developmental psychologist Lev Vygotsky wrote, "Internal and external action are inseparable: imagination, interpretation, and will are internal processes in external action" (Vygotskiĭ, 1933, 16). Thus, you cannot change one without changing the other. As someone who studied childhood, Vygotsky observed that children's behavior is exclusively motivated by their environment (determinism). After noting that every perception is a stimulus to activity, Lev Vygotsky goes on to state that,

> Since a situation is always, psychologically, accessed through perception, and perception is not separated from affective and motor activity, it is understandable that with his consciousness so structured, the child cannot act otherwise than as constrained by the situation—or the field—in which he finds himself.
>
> (Vygotskiĭ, 1933, 12)

In other words, all our actions, including thoughts and emotions, are the product of lived situations that create the implicit rules governing what we must do.

But when children play, they change that environment to suit their needs. For example, during play a bundle of rags becomes a baby, and the child becomes a mother. As Vygotsky puts it, "In play, external things lose their motivating force" (Vygotskiĭ, 1933, 12). Thus, creative play is how children escape external determinism and exercise choice. Their actions are indirectly selected through imagination and interpretation. Because one is always connected to the other, the two realities (internal/external) are inseparable.

Turning to imaginative involvement in adults, I would like to extend Vygotsky's logic:

(A) A = All psychological behavior is a response to situational factors (determinism).
(B) B = All situational factors are subject to the psychology of perception.
(C) C = The psychology of perception includes a capacity for creative imagination (choice).

This is a logical syllogism, if A = B and B = C, then C = A! In other words, when we reimagine our lived experiences, we find an opportunity to mediate the thing that controls us. It is like a dog on a leash learning how to tell his master where to walk and how much time to take in getting there. Thus, we are victims of circumstance only to the extent that we fail to engage the unconscious processes of creative imagination or divergent problem solving.

In regard to the age-old debate over free will versus determinism, I believe this creation of an either-or dichotomy, in which all-or-nothing thinking prevails, lacks relevance to the therapeutic endeavor. As Kirsch and Hyland (2017) have pointed out, science by necessity embraces *methodological determinism* because researchers are in the business of identifying causal chains. Conversely, most religions and governmental systems of justice embrace the concept of free will because these institutions are in the business of holding individuals accountable for their actions. However, therapists are in the business of caring for human consciousness, which involves supporting certain vital subjective experiences, such as hope/opportunity, meaning/purpose, and freedom/choice. In contrast to free will, *choice* is not a cosmological theory of being but rather a psychological experience.

When seeking to exercise choice within the framework of temporal reality, a legitimate task in psychotherapy is not only to change the client's future but also the subjective experience of the past. When changing the past, you change expectations for the future. Conversely, when you have the client imagine a new future and then bring memories from the past to consciousness, these memories are automatically modified and laid back down into long-term storage in a revised form.

This neurobiological process is not optional. It occurs regardless of whether it is utilized as a therapeutic strategy. The same is true of priming and suggestion. These are inherent to human interaction and therefore occur in all forms of therapy. The difference is that some therapists are trained to utilize these processes towards productive ends, while others deny their existence and perilously underestimate the scope of their influence.

Chapter 7 Key Points

- People problem solve more effectively when primed to reimagine the past.
- Memory is continually reconstructed—it is a creative process.

- A damaged sense of self can be repaired by altering the past or altering the future—a change in one automatically changes the other.
- Attending to new situational details counter-regulates emotional states leading to new emotions and new problem-solving behavior.
- We are victims of circumstance only to the extent that we fail to engage unconscious processes of creative imagination and play.

References

Arntz, Arnoud. 2012. "Imagery Rescripting as a Therapeutic Technique: Review of Clinical Trials, Basic Studies, and Research Agenda:" *Journal of Experimental Psychopathology* 3 (2): 189–208. doi:10.5127/jep.024211.

Bandura, Albert. 2000. "Exercise of Human Agency Through Collective Efficacy." *Current Directions in Psychological Science* 9 (3): 75–78. doi:10.1111/1467-8721.00064.

Brewin, Chris R. 2018. "Memory and Forgetting." *Current Psychiatry Reports* 20: 1–8. doi:10.1007/s11920-018-0950-7.

Coyle, Joseph T. 1997. *Memory Distortion: How Minds, Brains, and Societies Reconstruct the Past.* Boston, MA: Harvard University Press.

Driskell, James E., Carolyn Copper, and Aidan Moran. 1994. "Does Mental Practice Enhance Performance?" *Journal of Applied Psychology* 79 (4): 481–492. doi:10.1037/0021-9010.79.4.481.

Erickson, Milton H., and Ernest L. Rossi. 1979. *Hypnotherapy: An Exploratory Casebook.* Har/Cas edition. New York: Irvington Pub.

Erickson, Milton H., and Ernest Lawrence Rossi. 1989. *The February Man: Evolving Consciousness and Identity in Hypnotherapy.* New York: Brunner/Mazel Publishers.

Frankl, Viktor E. 1946. *Man's Search for Meaning.* 1st ed. New York: Pocket Books.

Galinsky, Adam D., and Gordon B. Moskowitz. 2000. "Counterfactuals as Behavioral Primes: Priming the Simulation Heuristic and Consideration of Alternatives." *Journal of Experimental Social Psychology* 36 (4): 384–409. doi:10.1006/jesp.1999.1409.

Garry, Maryanne, Charles G. Manning, Elizabeth F. Loftus, and Steven J. Sherman. 1996. "Imagination Inflation: Imagining a Childhood Event Inflates Confidence That It Occurred." *Psychonomic Bulletin & Review* 3 (2): 208–214. doi:10.3758/BF03212420.

Goulding, Mary McClure, and Robert L. Goulding. 1979. *Changing Lives Through Redecision Therapy.* New York: Grove Press.

James, William. (1890) 1927. *The Principles of Psychology*, Vol. I–II. New York: Henry Holt.

Janet, Pierre. 1894. "Histoire d'une idée fixe." *Review Philosophique de la France et de l'Etranger* 37: 121–168.

Jiang, Shui, Lynne Postovit, Annamaria Cattaneo, Elisabeth B. Binder, and Katherine J. Aitchison. 2019. "Epigenetic Modifications in Stress Response Genes Associated With Childhood Trauma." *Frontiers in Psychiatry* 10: 1–19. doi:10.3389/fpsyt.2019.00808.

Kirsch, Irving, and Michael E. Hyland. 2017. "Methodological Determinism and the Free Will Hypothesis." *Psychology of Consciousness: Theory, Research, and Practice* 4 (3): 321–323. doi:10.1037/cns0000135.

Lacan, Jacques, and Jeffrey Mehlman. 1987. "Introduction to the Names-of-the-Father Seminar." *October* 40: 81–95. doi:10.2307/778344.

Loftus, Elizabeth F., and Jacqueline E. Pickrell. 1995. "The Formation of False Memories." *Psychiatric Annals* 25 (12): 720–725. doi:10.3928/0048-5713-19951201-07.

Lynn, Steven Jay, Abigail Matthews, and Sean Barnes. 2012. "Hypnosis and Memory: From Bernheim to the Present." In *Handbook of Imagination and Mental Simulation*, edited by Keith D. Markman, William M. P. Klein, and Julie A. Suhr, 103–118. New York: Psychology Press.

Meichenbaum, Donald. 2014. "Don Meichenbaum Interviewed by Dan Short." *The Milton H. Erickson Foundation Newsletter* 34 (1): 1, 20–22. https://www.erickson-foundation.org/download/newsletters/Vol-34-No-1.pdf.

Peetz, Johanna, and Anne E. Wilson. 2008. "The Temporally Extended Self: The Relation of Past and Future Selves to Current Identity, Motivation, and Goal Pursuit." *Social and Personality Psychology Compass* 2 (6): 2090–2106. doi:10.1111/j.1751-9004.2008.00150.x.

Prince, Morton. 1912. *The Unconscious: The Fundamentals of Human Personality Normal and Abnormal.* New York: Macmillan.

Ross, Michael, and Anne Wilson. 2001. "Constructing and Appraising Past Selves." In *Memory, Brain, and Belief*, edited by Daniel L. Schacter and Elaine Scarry, 231–258. Boston, MA: Harvard University Press.

Rothermund, Klaus. 2011. "Counter-Regulation and Control-Dependency: Affective Processing Biases in the Service of Action Regulation." *Social Psychology* 42 (1): 56–66. doi:10.1027/1864-9335/a000043.

Sanna, Lawrence J. 2000. "Mental Simulation, Affect, and Personality: A Conceptual Framework." *Current Directions in Psychological Science* 9 (5): 168–173. doi:10.1111/1467-8721.00086.

Schwager, Susanne, and Klaus Rothermund. 2013. "Counter-Regulation Triggered by Emotions: Positive/Negative Affective States Elicit Opposite Valence Biases in Affective Processing." *Cognition and Emotion* 27 (5): 839–855. doi:10.1080/02699931.2012.750599.

Scoboria, Alan, Kimberley A. Wade, D. Stephen Lindsay, Tanjeem Azad, Deryn Strange, James Ost, and Ira E. Hyman. 2017. "A Mega-Analysis of Memory Reports from Eight Peer-Reviewed False Memory Implantation Studies." *Memory* 25 (2): 146–163. doi:10.1080/09658211.2016.1260747.

Smucker, Mervin R., Constance Dancu, Edna B. Foa, and Jan L. Niederee. 1995. "Imagery Rescripting: A New Treatment for Survivors of Childhood Sexual Abuse Suffering From Posttraumatic Stress." *Journal of Cognitive Psychotherapy* 9 (1): 3–17. doi:10.1891/0889-8391.9.1.3.

Tulving, Endel, and Fergus I. M. Craik. 2005. *The Oxford Handbook of Memory*. New York: Oxford University Press.

Vygotskiĭ, Lev Semenovich. 1933. "Igra i Ee Rol v Umstvennom Razvitii Rebenka." *Voprosy Psihologii* [*Problems of Psychology*] 12 (6): 62–76.

Wilson, Anne, and Michael Ross. 2003. "The Identity Function of Autobiographical Memory: Time Is on Our Side." *Memory* 11 (2): 137–149. doi:10.1080/741938210.

8 Mental Contrasting

This chapter seeks to answer the question: How does psychotherapy provide the means to pursue new ends without imposing an agenda? Of equal importance, How does the therapist provide sufficient yet open-ended structure so that the client is not left wallowing in indecision? The dilemma is that indigenous change (self-initiated) must be preceded by native goals (self-identified), but the type of self-empowered individual capable of formulating such goals rarely needs the assistance of a psychotherapist. Rather, those seeking mental health assistance are often demoralized and not certain which goals they should pursue.

This emphasis on client-selected goals was a defining aspect of the psychotherapy of Milton Erickson. He refused to impose his goals upon the will of the client. Instead, Erickson often used future-progression to transport the client into a desired future, using hypnosis to make it feel like a lived experience. We now know that attention to one's imagined future naturally evokes goal-oriented thinking and emotional concern for achieving those outcomes—a budding sense of ownership and responsibility.

Any exercise of foresight contains two subtextual questions: "What do I want?" and "How will I get it?" If that future is mentally simulated, then this virtual reality shows us what it means to fulfill our goals and what is needed to avoid the threat of failure. Because temporal reality is circular, this exercise creates an implicit contrast between the pain of past failures and the desire for future success. As Erickson puts it:

> You know, one of the most informative aspects of human behavior is this matter of hindsight. Hindsight is so awfully important, and you wonder why you didn't use this knowledge based on hindsight in the form of foresight. How often have you said to yourself, "If I had only known things would work out this way! I had all the data available to me beforehand, so why didn't I realize it would work out this way?" And in the practice of medicine and psychiatry, you need to speculate on how things are going to work out, and on how to use the available information.
>
> (Erickson and Rossi, 1984, 196)

DOI: 10.4324/9781003127208-8

Erickson emphasized the importance of eliciting involvement in an imagined future at the outset of therapy. This use of virtual reality to evaluate decisions and choices was in keeping with his insistence on placing the burden of responsibility for change on the shoulders of the client (Erickson, 1964). While teaching Jay Haley, Erickson argued that the act of securing a commitment to change is one of the first things done in the process of psychotherapy (Erickson and Haley, 1985).

This reminds me of a frequent admonition from one of my earliest mentors, John Gladfelter. At the time, nearly thirty years ago, I worked with court-ordered domestic violence offenders, a clientele for whom the motivation to engage in introspective work is typically low. As I struggled with how to best assist my clients, Gladfelter would caution me, "Never work harder than the client." In other words, it was my responsibility to inspire responsibility in the people I wished to help.

The worst way to go about this would be to lecture the client, saying, "You have to want to change. I can't make your life better for you!" I hope I never said such a thing. But imagine if I had. What would a court-ordered person, who is being forced into therapy, have thought to himself? It makes me wince at the thought.

A more effective approach is to appeal to automatic, future-oriented, imaginative capabilities that exist in every individual. This is the natural birthplace of goal-oriented thought. As I learned while still a neophyte therapist, if I said to my domestic violence client, "What are you most unhappy about?", he would always give me an honest answer (the same is true for teenagers mandated to therapy by their parents).

For example, the client population I served would often say,

> I am tired of being treated like shit by others. I don't want police in my home or judges telling me what to do. I don't want to work hard all day long just to come home and have my wife yell at me and my kids ignore me.

Surprisingly, this type of reply is fertile ground for planting the seeds of responsibility. All that is required is a future-oriented perspective. To achieve this, I would ask,

> When you come home, what would you like to see? Where would you like your wife and kids to be? Living at a women's shelter? Or, greeting you at the door? Do you want them to be smiling at you and glad that you are there? How would you like them to honestly feel about you returning home?

These questions evoke a great deal of mental simulation. To answer any of my questions, the client must automatically construct an imagined future.

If he is able to do so, I will see an emerging capacity for responsibility in his reply. For example, often these men would say to me,

> I would like to have my wife and kids greet me at the door when I come home. I would like for them to be happy to see me. I work hard to pay the bills. I would like everyone to appreciate what I do for them.

That mental image will start to define an emerging set of implicit goals.

Often, my next question would be,

> Are your current strategies working? Is your anger getting the outcomes you want? ... Think about the last time you yelled at your wife. What did you see on her face? How did she act afterwards? What did the children do? Did they run and hide, or did they stick around and try to defend their mother?

This is the point at which a client with a weakened ego might resort to defensive behaviors, such as using blame, denial, or distraction. Therefore, I found it crucial to engage my clients with respect, as intellectual beings capable of important problem-solving abilities. This was achieved by asking questions such as: "What do you think is the biggest obstacle to your success?" or "What do you need to be able to change in order to get the outcomes you want?"

Whatever the answer might have been, it was met with my enthusiastic support and willingness to collaborate on that self-identified goal (indigenous change).

8.1 Envisioning a Compelling Future

The next technique we will learn is similar to reimagining in its use of mental simulation and prefactual information; however, the emphasis is shifted from self-appraisal (how memories and expectations can redefine sense of self) to external achievements (how personal goals and plans influence outcomes). This goal-oriented means of activating unconscious resources is currently studied under the terminology of *mental contrasting* (goals vs. obstacles). It is the first step in a two-step methodology that is evidence-based and process-oriented (Oettingen and Kappes, 2009).

When you ask any client "What do you want to see happening in your future?", the answer helps establish the idea that it is they who must take responsibility for both the problems they face and the outcomes they wish to produce. When you next ask about the obstacles that he or she sees standing in the way of progress, then the motivation to change behavior is enriched with intellectual problem-solving—without requiring conscious effort. In other words, mental contrasting is essentially a means of consolidating goal commitment as an unconscious process.

It is important to understand that a process-oriented approach to psychotherapy does not impose society's goals and standards on its clientele (we have educational, religious, and justice systems for that job). Just as importantly, psychotherapists should resist the temptation to impose goals derived from their own personal life experience or from the theoretical models of mental health by which they have been indoctrinated.

In unconscious process work, problem-solving goals automatically emerge from within and from beyond the margin of conscious awareness. In this expansive universe of images and simulated events, there is often a failure of words to adequately describe the meaning of newly-identified needs. Thus, we should not become overly concerned with how the client states his or her goals. Furthermore, the means for achieving these indigenous goals is not entirely decided by conscious awareness.

This brings us to the second step in mental contrasting, which is to identify how the obstacles to success will be overcome (implementation intentions). As shown by Gollwitzer and Sheeran (2006), this extra step increases the likelihood that goal-oriented behavior will be enacted without conscious thought. Essentially, implementation intentions detail when, where, and how goal-oriented action will occur. The strategy uses if-then plans to link a situational trigger to a response. The "if" part of the contingency plan identifies an anticipated obstacle. Next, the "then" part sets up a goal-directed response for automatic activation when the obstacle is encountered. When conscious planning is used to establish automatic responses, the result is greater consistency between explicit and implicit problem-solving behavior (the same goal is being processed consciously and unconsciously). I can illustrate the dynamic nature of this approach using a recent case example.

A long-term client had attended 37 sessions with me, spread across eight years. He entered therapy emotionally hardened, narcissistically closed-off, and unavailable for human intimacy (his only close relationship was with his dog). His police background, in a tactical unit that pursued dangerous drug cartel members, put him in the position of needing to be able to kill others without experiencing emotional distress. However, during his time in therapy, he had significantly increased both his humanity and his need for human connection.

We never really discussed his childhood. Even so, it was clear that it contained darkness. Without the experience of secure attachment, the decision to allow himself to emotionally need someone was a tremendous leap of faith, yet he took that plunge. He moved in with a woman whom he had known for years and had come to love deeply. But he was having difficulty with the demands of the relationship and his ongoing struggle against historical feelings of inadequacy. His automatic tendency was to withdraw by ending the relationship.

As he explained it to me,

> Dr. Short, I do not want to become angry or insecure when I am around her. But F-CK! She keeps finding fault with all that I am trying to do for her. I spent the entire day working on her house. I replaced her refrigerator for the second time. The first one wasn't good enough. I leveled the refrigerator doors for a third time. I fixed the pop-up heads on the sprinklers. I painted the bedroom. I have worked my ass off, and all she can do is find fault. I understand she grew up on the farm, and that is just how her family talks. It's all about work and doing things to a standard of perfection. But f-ck! I can feel myself starting to get angry, and that is not good.

I assumed he might want me to help him figure out how to get a little more validation from the woman he loved. But that was not the direction he took the conversation. Instead, he explained,

> I need to learn how to become more self-sufficient. I don't need my ego becoming dependent on what she says. … We had a talk about this, and she was honestly concerned about how she should talk to me so that I'm not getting my feelings hurt. But she doesn't need to be walking around on eggshells so that I can feel okay about myself. She needs to be able to be herself and me be fine with it.

As I reflected inwardly, privately asking myself whether I am holding myself to a high enough standard in my own marriage, he looked me in the eyes and asked,

> How do I make myself care less about what others think? Instead, I want to be able to make myself feel okay with who I am. I do not want to be addicted to other people's praise or affirmations. I used to do crazy shit so that others would admire me more than anyone else in the room. I don't want to be that guy anymore.

Knowing that he had impressive knowledge of military history, I framed my response in those terms. I said,

> There is a strategy that they teach soldiers about how to resist interrogations in case they are captured by the enemy. I wish I knew more about this because it would help you make yourself more immune to outside influence. It has something to do with not viewing the captor as an authority figure … instead referencing in your imagination the commander back home, seeking to stay consistent with a goal that you know would please him or make him proud. … I cannot remember his name, but it was a strategy used by a famous pilot shot down during the Vietnam war.

At this point, my client's face lit up. He said I must be talking about James Stockdale, who was a Navy vice-admiral and one of the most highly decorated officers in the history of the US Navy. After his plane was shot down over Vietnam in 1965, Stockdale told himself that he was leaving the world of technology and entering the world of Epictetus (50–135 AD). My client explained, "That is who Stockdale consulted during his captivity. During seven-and-a-half years of captivity, Stockdale spent four of those years in solitary confinement, which meant he needed this type of stimulation to keep himself sane."

My client told me that Stockdale learned from Epictetus how to care about those things that are within our control and just accept the rest. As more information began to become active in his unconscious working memory, my client suddenly quoted Marcus Aurelius, "It doesn't hurt me unless I interpret what has happened as harmful to me, and I can choose not to." This meant that at some level he had already formulated a future narrative of consulting Marcus Aurelius the same way Stockdale had consulted Epictetus. No doubt, his creative unconscious was exploring numerous future scenarios.

Feeling that I still owed him some sort of formal advice, I seized upon his unconscious plan and made it explicit, saying,

> The next time you feel criticized or find yourself needing external approval, envision Marcus Aurelius watching you and speaking to you about your accomplishments or your mistakes. This way you meet your human need for external validation, but really it is coming from inside of you—you will be depending on your inner strength rather than feeling that you need to control others.

He responded with great enthusiasm, "I love it! I know exactly what to do. This makes perfect sense to me." In order to make his implementation of this strategy automatic, I told him, "Think about it a while with your eyes closed. See yourself using this strategy. Notice what is happening."

Sitting with his eyes closed, he spent several minutes in deep meditation. When he opened his eyes, he smiled from ear to ear and said, "This is really good. Can we end early? I want to write this down and think about it some more." He did not want to discuss anything else because he wished to remain fully absorbed in his visions of him implementing this strategy in the future with different people and in different settings.

One of the interesting features of this case is that, as the therapist, I never suggested that my client should somehow change his thoughts or his behavior. I did not teach any new concepts. I did not identify a problem or a solution. He came to therapy with the goal of increasing his emotional self-regulation and preserving his emotional self-sufficiency. He wanted to treat someone special to him with extraordinary kindness and generosity. All that I did was to help him imagine a future-oriented context in which he was able to successfully implement these goals.

8.2 Focusing on Success

Sometimes a student of psychotherapy will ask me, "How do you make the changes that occur in therapy permanent?" This question does not come from a growth mindset. Changes that are permanent result in rigidity and a loss of adaptive capability. This reminds me of the famous quote from Heraclitus (535–475 BC), "You could not step twice into the same river." As Plato explained, "It is not the same river, and he is not the same man." If Heraclitus is correct that everything changes, then so must our goals, our solutions, and even the definition of what constitutes a problem.

Therefore, it is not the behavioral or intellectual product of a problem-solving endeavor that has the greatest value. Rather, it is the process of strengthening one's own problem-solving abilities that matters most. The act of problem solving is how we manifest self-efficacy and choice. Without problem solving, everything we might hope for is either predestined or impossible.

Any attempt to use reason to find information that is missing is a problem to be solved. Any attempt to create something new and valuable is a problem to be solved. And, any attempt to choose between alternatives is a problem to be solved. Even as we sleep, the unconscious mind explores, through dreaming, the formulation of problems and solutions relative to the day's activities and any related history. If problem solving is the daily air that we breathe, then good therapy is something that expands our lung capacity.

With unconscious process work, the top priority is not to teach the client to engage in effortful attempts to establish goals and identify obstacles to overcome, but rather to learn how to do this automatically. When using foresight to effectively organize behavior, we want the client to be able to declare, "It's just who I am." I say it this way because once a behavior passes from conscious effort to unconscious automation, we tend to embrace it as a native feature of our identity.

For example, when a potential friend asks, "Why do you push people away?", the typical response would be, "That is just who I am." Hardly anyone stops to reflect on the original goal that established the behavior. If they did, it might sound something like,

> Well, as a child I grew up in a military family, which meant we were moving every two years. By the age of twelve, I could no longer stand the pain of losing best friends and having to start over as a stranger in school. Needing to somehow protect my heart, I decided to no longer form close friendships. Having become deeply accustomed to this goal, it is now habitual.

For this person's life to change, his (unconscious) goals need to change. And for that to happen, he merely needs to be asked, "What would you like to see yourself gaining from your relationships with others and what is standing in your way?" Research shows that this mental contrast will lead to new goal formation.

To facilitate greater realization of one's own innate goodness, the therapist needs to aim for indigenous change, what Erickson described as naturalistic change. But growth does not occur without the presence of challenging goals. This explains why researchers Locke and Latham (2002) found that statements such as "Just do your best" do not lead to increased problem-solving ability. Rather, the client is invited to exercise choice by envisioning a future that represents a step forward towards some improved version of self. If I wish to help someone grow, then I use the question recommended by Locke and Latham, "What more can you do?" This open-ended question leads to an unconscious search for unrealized potentials.

When people expect to fail, they do not engage effortfully. Sometimes this is called self-sabotage or self-handicapping. These terms infer that a person has somehow become their own adversary, but that is not the best way to view it. There is less speculation if we simply acknowledge a divide between goals pursued consciously and those pursued outside of awareness. Sometimes, the goals we pursue through conscious intention are overly ambitious. That is when it is helpful to use mental contrasting to bridge the divide.

For example, if a woman (who is in an abusive relationship) declares, "I am leaving the relationship! I will not allow him to talk me into returning," then I will want to make certain this is realistic. In this type of situation, I will ask the client, "How easy is it for you to see yourself doing this? What is the probability that you will follow through with your plan?" If the client responds, "There is at least a 25% chance," then I point out that 50% is nothing more than random chance. Then I explain, "You are telling me there is a 75% chance that this goal is too big for you." I do not want the client to set herself up for failure. It will have a negative impact on her expectations for future goals. And, it might make her feel too ashamed to return to therapy.

I protect my clients from failure by asking, "*What more can you do* that has at least an 80% chance of success?" To have the same question processed at unconscious levels, I can add the question, "What can you see yourself doing?" What has been found in research by Oettingen and colleagues (2001) is that for mental contrasting to produce positive results (for a person to commit to a goal and strive to achieve this desired future) the expectation of success needs to be high.

If I refrain from advising the client on what her next, small step should be, it helps reduce the risk of me accidentally insulting the client. This is one of the key advantages to using mental contrasting. As found in research conditions, when a person is asked to envision a desirable and feasible future, which is then contrasted with a negative outcome, people not only become more resolute in their goal striving but are also less affected when confronted with strong negative feedback.

Researchers argue that by energizing people to realize their wishes, form plans, and commit to them in line with their subjective probabilities of success, negative feedback can actually increase the optimistic outlook! If the feedback provides meaningful information, the person can include it in their vision of future success. Putting this subjective reaction to words might sound something like, "I'm so glad you told me that. Now I am even more likely to succeed." As demonstrated by Oettingen and Kappes (2009), this positive reaction to negative feedback does not occur for those who have low expectations for success.

While trying to conceptualize the value of mental contrasting, keep in mind that it produces more than the eye will ever see. Mental contrasting has been shown experimentally to activate goals at multiple levels, with some of the goals being explicit and others implicit. This is in keeping with nearly three decades of research showing that goals can be activated unconsciously, even as people pursue other conscious goals, and the activated goals are then pursued outside of conscious awareness (Kruglanski, 1996; Bargh, 1990). It is important for people to describe their problems and develop a coherent narrative about their past. But these activities are not therapeutic unless they lead to some vision of the future. If people are not invited to dream about their future, then there is a failure to engage unconscious goal activation and the emotional-motivational abilities that come with it. The brain is an organ that is designed to transform thought into reality, but to do so we must produce a task that activates its multi-systemic functions. Mental contrasting appears to be one way of doing this.

8.3 Planning Automatic Behavior

Most of us have heard the proverb, "the road to hell is paved with good intentions." This saying is meant to highlight the false sense of accomplishment that comes with having good intentions but no plan of action. When seeking to measure how wide this proverbial road is, Webb and Sheeran (2006) found that intentions account for only 28% of the variance, thus intentions are relatively poor predictors of future behavior.

Returning to the concept of self-handicapping, if a young student tells his parents, "Don't worry, I'll study for the exam," then there is cause for concern. Their child may honestly have good intentions (the road to hell), which means that theoretically there is a 72% probability that he will not be ready for that test.

Ironically, the greater the student's fear of failure, the more likely he is to avoid the intended behavior (not study until midnight on the night before the test). It is as if the person has the conscious intention to succeed even as he unconsciously prepares for failure. The subsequent failure then leads to more self-reassuring intentions, "Next time, I will really study hard," which produce no better outcomes. This cycle can have endless repetitions. So, what does one do?

One strategy is to send the child to a hypnotherapist. In this setting, a skilled practitioner would use deep imaginative involvement to create emotionally compelling mental simulations. Each of these will be future oriented, such as a vision of the child proudly announcing to his parents that he made good grades on the test, sharing the good news with an encouraging football coach, bragging to kids who teased him for being dumb, or whatever matters most to the student. This helps strategically activate unconscious motivation. Next, the hypnotherapist will have the child see all the different obstacles that stand in the way of him realizing that highly desirable outcome and how he will overcome them. To help initiate solution-oriented behavior, a post-hypnotic suggestion will be provided. For example, the hypnotherapist might say, "When you come home from school each day, you will feel a new sense of joy as you study and realize you are becoming smarter and smarter."

Other obstacles faced by this student might include excessive pressure from a hostile, overly controlling parent. If this were the case, the posthypnotic suggestion would need to be a little more complex. The therapist might say,

> The next time your step dad is harassing you and telling you that you should make better grades, you will really teach him a lesson. For one test you will study enough to make an A. Then, on the next test, you will make any grade you choose to make. That way, you get to show how successful you can be whenever you want. And you do not have to make all Fs to prove this point. It will be much more satisfying to add in some As as well.

Though the statement is multifaceted, it is still the same basic formula that is used in all post-hypnotic suggestions, "*if X, then Y*" (if your stepdad harasses you, then you will teach him a lesson). We should recognize that this is an implementation strategy.

Post-hypnotic suggestion enables automatic action by assigning control of one's goal-directed thoughts, feelings, and behaviors to specific situational cues rather than conscious intentionality. What we now know from research outside of hypnosis (no trance involved) is that the mental act of linking a critical situation to an intended behavior in the form of an *if-then* plan leads to automatic action. The resulting response to the critical situation is swift, efficient, and does not require conscious intent. Thus, the primary difference between post-hypnotic suggestion and unconscious process work is that traditionally in hypnosis it is the hypnotherapist who formulates the *if-then* plan. With unconscious process work the planning is indigenous—it is formulated by the client.

Thanks to the work of Peter Gollwitzer and colleagues (2006), there is a growing body of evidence that convincingly demonstrates the importance of enriching people's intentions with specific, feasible plans of action. This is what separates daydreaming (satisfying the desire for change by imagining that it could occur) from achievement motivation (delaying emotional gratification until the goal is reached). What Gollwitzer has found is that automatic action control can be achieved strategically by forming implementation intentions that follow the formula, "If Situation *X* is encountered, then I will perform Behavior *Y*." By using emotionally meaningful imagery, which includes a concrete response, a strong mental link is created between a specified future situation and the anticipated goal-directed response. This process does not depend on hypnotic suggestion but rather on the client's implicit ability to exercise foresight.

Gollwitzer's basic message is that to succeed in solving challenging problems, people only need to furnish their goals with relevant plans that spell out in an *if-then* manner how the task at hand is to be performed. This exercise creates a different mindset, as there is an intellectual transition from "what I want" to "how can I?" Gollwitzer refers to this transition as crossing the Rubicon, meaning that, just as for Julius Caesar, there is no turning back once the boundary is crossed.

When having a client envision implementation intentions, it is helpful to include as much topography as possible: when will you do this, where will you do it, and how will you do it? This helps strategically prepare automatic responses to critical situations. What Gollwitzer and colleagues (2006) learned while testing the "Rubicon model" is that planning does not come as naturally to people as setting goals. This helps explain why the road to hell is so wide. Recent research demonstrates that goal attainment is substantially improved when people are explicitly instructed to furnish their goals with plans. Thus, planning serves as a self-regulation strategy for goal attainment.

Another interesting finding from Gollwitzer and Brandstätter (1997) is that the more difficult it is to initiate the goal-directed behavior, the more useful it is to establish implementation intentions. When faced with easy goals planning is more cumbersome than productive. However, when conducting psychotherapy we should expect to be confronting challenging problems. If this is not the case, then the therapist might be focused on the wrong set of goals—a mere distraction from the goals that are linked to shame or deep pain.

As most of us would expect, implementation intentions are ineffective when they do not serve a valued goal. Therefore, mental contrasting is always the first step in the process. Clients must first envision themselves living a future that has great emotional value. As an outside observer, the therapist can easily see if there is an emotional reaction. When the image of the desired future emerges automatically, it is a non-volitional act of will.

A second act of willing is achieved by making *if-then* plans that are intuitive or automatic. This can be achieved using any therapeutic protocol that results in the surrender of conscious control. What this looks like in practical terms is any situation that primes the individual to forecast future obstacles and automatically envision a response that is most likely to overcome the obstacle. This planning can be achieved using a hypnotherapeutic protocol, free-association, imagery, role play, writing a letter, meditation/prayer, or any cultural scheme that best meets the client's emotional needs.

It is the type of approach we saw occur in the case study with the man who was trying to be the best version of himself within a maturing relationship. Though I can make educated guesses, I did not know for certain why he wanted to become entirely emotionally self-sufficient. Furthermore,

I did not know how he should plan to achieve such a thing. But I did have enough knowledge about my client's lifetime of learning to know the direction to point him so he could access the information he needed to construct his *if-then* strategies.

To sum up this process of planning automatic behavior, after the person has envisioned a compelling future (implicit goal-setting), then the next step is to imagine the process of achieving this outcome step by step. This is done in great enough detail to gain foresight into when, where, and how the person will need to act. By formulating this plan in an *if-then* mental representation, the situational trigger becomes easier to recognize in the environment. As shown in research, linking the situation to a goal-directed response creates a strong mental association that allows people to initiate the specified response automatically as soon as the critical situation is encountered. This link produces the planned behavior even in the absence of conscious intent to act. As Gollwitzer and Sheeran (2006) point out, this planning helps people overcome problems of conscious self-regulation, such as procrastination, distraction, or overextending one's self.

8.4 Therapeutic Immediacy

For William James, practice is one of the most essential components in the change process. Whether the change is behavioral or emotional, James believed that new patterns must be solidified through activation and repetition. As James (1916) states:

> A tendency to act only becomes effectively ingrained in us in proportion to the uninterrupted frequency with which the actions actually occur, and the brain "grows" to their use. When a resolve or a fine glow of feeling is allowed to evaporate without bearing practical fruit, it is worse than a chance lost: it works so as positively to hinder future resolutions and emotions from taking the normal path to discharge.
> (70)

In other words, whenever people fail to act on their intentions, the initiative will quickly decay. James argued that by setting an intention and then not acting on it at the first opportunity, the person nullifies the motivation to act while also conditioning him or herself to repeat avoidance behavior. That is why James believed that when the goal-oriented thought appears, you must act immediately.

Similarly, immediacy has great relevance to therapy. Therapeutic immediacy is any attempt to close the gap between a new therapeutic goal and the opportunity to implement goal-seeking behavior. If a client laments, "I need to say these things to my mother, don't I?", then I might reply, "Yes. Do you have a cell phone handy?" If the client wishes to have privacy, then I leave my office. This is therapeutic immediacy. Without it, the client will return a week later with no phone call to her mother.

The motivation to act is always strongest when the client is sitting in front of his or her therapist. After the meeting ends, every hour that passes sees a significant reduction in this motivation. Feelings change once the client is no longer looking into the eyes of his or her therapist. Experience suggests that only two days after the session, this motivation will have evaporated. It is only the night before the next appointment that the lost motivation comes thundering back.

Thus, clients need to do something in relation to their problem, preferably the moment a desire for change is expressed. It is extremely useful for the therapist to have some repertoire of experiential exercises so that clients can engage immediately in a goal-oriented task. Even a small, symbolic gesture, completed in the office, tends to solidify the subjective experience of commitment. For example, if the client who needs to talk to her mother tells me that she is not ready, then we can spend some time discussing the obstacles that stand in her way. This is the beginning of contingency planning that will automatically move her from complaining about her problem to doing something about it. Next, I can help her envision overcoming those obstacles. This is where mental rehearsal serves a vital purpose.

Because imagination can establish new neural connections, as does empirical reality, it becomes a convenient means for creating experiences during which new stimulus-response pairings can be achieved. Milton Erickson seems to have capitalized on this fact by using *hypnotic rehearsal* (trance, imagination, and imagery) to have patients practice new behaviors. While using what he called the *rehearsal method*, Erickson might have a person hypnotically experience themselves implementing the solution to their problem at least a dozen times, perhaps more. The impact created by this virtual reality is made greater through the incorporation of detail. Making reference to his work with a specific patient, Erickson (1952) explains,

> After exploration of the underlying causes of her problem, the next step in therapy was to outline in great detail, with her help, the exact course of activity that she would have to follow to free herself from past rigidly established habitual patterns of behavior.
>
> (257)

Before a patient would leave Erickson's office, he or she would have already begun the process of establishing a new habit. The same dynamic is achieved, without trance, by simply asking the client to imagine him or herself implementing the solution. To ensure that unconscious process work is achieved, the implementation intentions need to emerge automatically from the client's creative unconscious, or as Erickson states, the client helps determine "the exact course of activity."

This idea of using imaginative involvement to repeat problem-solving behavior multiple times, in multiple settings, under multiple conditions reminds me of a quote from Bruce Lee, "I fear not the man who has learned a 1,000 techniques, but the man who has practiced one technique a thousand times." Similarly, another world champion martial arts fighter and close friend of mine, Richard Pogue, once said to me,

> You do not need much conscious awareness to fight. Not if you have practiced enough times. I once saw a fighter get knocked unconscious and still use his arms and legs to apply a choke hold. It took a while for everyone to realize that he was unconscious.

Just as we see in the literature on flow states of consciousness, with enough rehearsal a person will not need to engage conscious control to execute their implementation strategy at the highest level of personal performance.

8.5 Bridging and Transfer Effects

In Chapter 5 we saw how important analogies can be for refining unconscious knowledge. This is especially true for mental contrasting. Although it seems as if goal-oriented thinking must always focus on the future, we need to remember that the psychological relationship between the future and the past is circular, not linear. There is an interdependency between temporal dimensions—the future can change our experience of the past, and the past determines what we are able to see in the future. Any goal-oriented thought about the future, when infused with accomplishments from the past, will attain greater dimensionality both in terms of implicit understanding as well as emotional significance. And, the use of analogy instantly bridges the space between the future and the past.

For example, if a woman is proud of the fact that at a young age she packed her bags and moved to a new country all on her own, then that accomplishment is psychological capital that can be invested in other problem-solving endeavors. If she were to come to therapy many years later feeling trapped in an abusive relationship, then a nice question to ask would be, "What is keeping you from packing your bags once again?"

A lot happens with this question. First, it creates a mental contrast between the less desirable reality of feeling trapped versus the freedom to leave a bad situation. Secondly, implementation intentions are suggested because packing one's bags is literally a piece of the plan to leave. Since the question is open ended, there is space for her to spontaneously identify all the other steps that need to be taken. Finally, the analogy (moving from one country to another = leaving a bad relationship) produces transfer effects so that the internal lessons she learned from her past accomplishment can be transferred over to the current task. As demonstrated by Gollwitzer (1999) the benefits of a problem-solving mindset will transfer to other tasks and other life domains.

By utilizing transfer effects during mental contrasting, therapists can help clients make progress in other domains where expectations for obtaining the desired outcome remain low. For example, consider the school teacher who comes to therapy for help with her biological children, who will not listen to her. While working with such a client, my first question was, "When the school principal visits your classroom, what does he say?" Her proud reply was, "He congratulates me on having such a well-managed classroom." My next question was, "What would your home look like if you manage it the same way you do your classroom?" This is an invitation for mental contrasting and indigenous change—versus me telling her how to make things better. After I asked this question, she was initially at a loss for words. My guess is that at some level she was processing the image of her home looking and sounding more like her classroom. Then she replied, "I never thought about using my training at home. It's so strange that you can have all of these wonderful skills and not use any of them." After I helped her further envision the plan for using her teaching skills at home, no further therapy was needed.

This problem-solving strategy is referred to as bridging—using a past achievement as an analogy to better understand an immediate challenge. These transfer effects, from one task to another or across domains, are not automatic. It seems that conscious awareness is required. However, once the connection is made, unconscious processing will take over as expectations of success are drawn from relevant experiential memories and implicit learning. As with other forms of mental contrasting, bridging helps clients better tolerate initial setbacks or negative feedback. Furthermore, it is the surest method of building self-efficacy. Whether conscious or not, at some level the client says to him or herself, "If I did it once before, then I can do it again."

Chapter 8 Key Points

- Asking clients to imagine a preferred future helps establish unconscious, indigenous goals. Readiness is enhanced when clients imagine themselves overcoming obstacles along the way.
- Motivation and resiliency to negative feedback are increased by focusing on positive outcomes (that clients consider attainable) in contrast to negative outcomes.
- Creating implementation intentions—planning where, when, and how goal-oriented action will occur ("if X occurs, then I will do Y")—increases automatic implementation.
- Use mental rehearsal to strengthen implementation: imagining the new behavior multiple times in multiple settings and under multiple conditions.
- Use former achievements to create a bridge to better understand immediate challenges.

References

Bargh, John A. 1990. "Goal and Intent: Goal-Directed Thought and Behavior Are Often Unintentional." *Psychological Inquiry* 1 (3): 248–251. doi:10.1207/s15327965pli0103_14.

Erickson, Milton H. 1952. "Deep Hypnosis and Its Induction." In *Collected Works of Milton H. Erickson, Volume 1: The Nature of Therapeutic Hypnosis*, edited by Ernest L. Rossi, Roxanna Erickson-Klein, and Kathryn Rossi, 229–260. Phoenix, AZ: Milton H. Erickson Foundation Press.

Erickson, Milton H. 1964. "The Burden of Responsibility in Effective Psychotherapy." *American Journal of Clinical Hypnosis* 6 (3): 269–271. doi:10.1080/00029157.1964.10402352.

Erickson, Milton H., and Jay Haley. 1985. *Conversations with Milton H. Erickson, M. D., Vol I: Changing Individuals*. 1st edition. San Diego, CA: Triangle Press.

Erickson, Milton H., and Ernest L. Rossi. 1984. *Life Reframing in Hypnosis*. Edited by Margaret O. Ryan. Har/Cas Edition. New York: Irvington Pub.

Gollwitzer, Peter M. 1999. "Deliberative versus Implemental Mindsets in the Control of Action." In *Dual-Process Theories in Social Psychology*, edited by Shelly Chaiken and Yaacov Trope, 403–422. New York: Guilford Press.

Gollwitzer, Peter M., and Veronika Brandstätter. 1997. "Implementation Intentions and Effective Goal Pursuit." *Journal of Personality and Social Psychology* 73 (1): 186–199.

Gollwitzer, Peter M., and Paschal Sheeran. 2006. "Implementation Intentions and Goal Achievement: A Meta-analysis of Effects and Processes." *Advances in Experimental Social Psychology* 38: 69–119. doi:10.1016/S0065-2601(06)38002–1.

James, William. (1916) 1925. *Talks To Teachers On Psychology; And To Students On Some Of Life's Ideals*. New York: Henry Holt. Project Gutenberg. http://www.gutenberg.org/ebooks/16287.

Kruglanski, Arie W. 1996. "Goals as Knowledge Structures." In *The Psychology of Action: Linking Cognition and Motivation to Behavior*, edited by P. M. Gollwitzer and J. A. Bargh, 599–618. New York: The Guilford Press.

Locke, Edwin A., and Gary P. Latham. 2002. "Building a Practically Useful Theory of Goal Setting and Task Motivation: A 35-Year Odyssey." *American Psychologist* 57 (9): 705–717. doi:10.1037/0003-066X.57.9.705.

Oettingen, Gabriele, and Andreas Kappes. 2009. "Mental Contrasting of the Future and Reality to Master Negative Feedback." In *Handbook of Imagination and Mental Simulation*, edited by Keith D. Markman, William M. P. Klein, and Julie A. Suhr, 395–412. New York: Psychology Press.

Oettingen, Gabriele, Hyeon-ju Pak, and Karoline Schnetter. 2001. "Self-Regulation of Goal-Setting: Turning Free Fantasies about the Future into Binding Goals." *Journal of Personality and Social Psychology* 80 (5): 736–753. doi:10.1037/0022-3514.80.5.736.

Webb, Thomas L., and Paschal Sheeran. 2006. "Does Changing Behavioral Intentions Engender Behavior Change?: A Meta-Analysis of the Experimental Evidence." *Psychological Bulletin* 132 (2): 249–268. doi:10.1037/0033-2909.132.2.249.

9 Incubated Cognition

The electrifying experience of profound insight is ancient—something that was initially attributed to divine intervention and summoned by prophets. By the tenth century, insight became the object of intentional practice, such as the Buddhist quest for vipaśyanā (Sanskrit for insight or "special-seeing"). In this spiritual context, insight is the experience of obtaining greater comprehension of the nature of reality.

When Freud (1900) chose insight as the central aim of psychotherapy, he limited its meaning to the revelation of individual psychology, during which content from the *id* (unconscious processes) is used to expand the *ego* (conscious reason). Insight continues to be pursued in psychoanalysis through self-observation, memory recovery, cognitive participation, and reconstruction in the context of affective reliving (catharsis). A central assumption is that insight is the result of a client-directed process that is therapeutic in itself (Neubauer, 1979).

A trade secret known to masters of psychotherapy is that when it comes to insight, the process of working to achieve it is equally as important as having a solution. As a novice therapist, I would sometimes blurt out a clever solution to a complex psychological dilemma only to have the client develop a spontaneous amnesia for my insight and then express disappointment that nothing had been achieved on that visit. Then, on their very next visit, these clients would come in excited about a compelling insight they had about their situation and then recite to me the same idea I had shared on the previous visit. After witnessing how important it was for the idea to first be processed by unconscious cognition, I had my own compelling insight, which was that solutions can be seeded to the unconscious (using the language devices described in Chapter 5), but before the idea can flourish in conscious awareness, it must germinate beneath the surface. While it is possible for therapists to share their point of view, this is not a viable substitute for embodied realities that emerge from the client's unconscious process work. As penned by Marshall McLuhan (1962, 246), "A point of view can be a dangerous luxury when substituted for insight and understanding."

As we progress from the Freudian idea of insight to a modern conceptualization, recognize that we are less interested in what is wrong with the

DOI: 10.4324/9781003127208-9

person than what the solution might be. When clients come to psychotherapy, they are struggling with what they feel to be impossible problems that are unresponsive to the solutions they know and understand. These types of problems require creative insight—not conscious analysis. Unfortunately, the more the client tries to focus effortful concentration on the problem, the more diminished his or her creative capacity will become—similar to "writer's block." Now, we have a neurological explanation for this phenomenon.

Cognitive neuroscientists Edward Bowden and Mark Jung-Beeman have observed that different types of problems require different types of mental processing (Bowden et al., 2005). Problems that require sequential conscious analysis are best handled by the brain's left hemisphere (logical thought). However, insight-oriented problems, which require access to remote associations and creativity, are best handled by the right hemisphere (unconscious thought), which has specialized neural cells with dendritic trees that are longer, more branched, and possess more dendritic spines—literally more capable of complex, far-reaching connections.

This fits with research by social psychologists Dijksterhuis and Meurs (2006), who have shown that unconscious thought is more divergent and associative (it makes lots of creative connections) than conscious thought. Furthermore, this implicit intellectual process benefits from an incubation period (when conscious examination of the problem is delayed for hours, days, or even weeks, this is known as an incubation period). Similarly, Jung-Beeman argues that effortful thought interferes with insight because focused concentration favors the left hemisphere, causing the right to become less active. Ironically, insight is not likely to occur until the person is helped to relax and focus his or her attention elsewhere (interview by Lehrer, 2012).

As used in this book, insight simply means progressing from a profound problem to a subjectively meaningful solution. When this occurs, new embodied understandings emerge in a way that alters one's experience of reality. An example of achieving insight following a brief incubation period can be observed in a case described by Erickson (1960) of a 50-year-old woman who came to his office for help with advanced Raynaud's Disease. She suffered extreme pain and sleep deprivation. Showing her hands to Erickson, she said, "I have got ulcerated fingers from lack of circulation to my hands. I have already had one finger amputated, and I expect I will have to have another amputation." She described her pain as being so intense that she could only sleep for one or two hours at a time.

Erickson responded by saying that he did not know much about treating Raynaud's Disease. He told her that if there was anything that could be done about this, her own "body learnings" would take care of the matter. He then taught her how to go into a trance during which he explained she had a tremendous amount of body learnings, the visceral abilities that we all accumulate over a lifetime of experience.

Erickson predicted that during the day her unconscious mind would be completely absorbed in correlating all her body learnings to use for her benefit.

Before going to bed, Erickson wanted her to sit in a chair and develop a state of profound relaxation. During that trance state she was to put all her learnings into action. After returning to normal waking awareness, she was to call Erickson.

The woman followed Erickson's instructions. Before bedtime she went into a trance. She called Erickson at 10:30 p.m. and in a trembling voice said,

> My husband is holding the phone because I am too weak to hold the receiver. I am scared! I can scarcely sit in the chair. I did exactly what you said. I sat in the chair and went into a trance and then all of a sudden, I started to get cold. I got colder and colder, just like when I was a little girl in Minnesota. I shivered all over for about twenty minutes. My teeth even chattered! Then suddenly the cold disappeared, and I began to get warm. I felt burning hot all over! Now I have developed a profound sense of physical relaxation and fatigue.

Erickson responded by saying, "Congratulations for teaching me how to handle this sort of a problem. Now go to bed and call me when you wake up." Erickson received the next call at 8:00 a.m. It was her first continuous night's sleep in over ten years.

Erickson explained this outcome saying, "I did not do anything other than to tell her to utilize, in her own way, her own special body learnings." Several months later he received a letter telling him that she had remained free of pain by using this method of capillary dilation in her arms, wrists, and hands. Each night, before she went to bed, she would alter the circulation of her blood so that she was able to achieve comfort in her hands and was therefore able to sleep through the night.

If we look at this case from a problem-solving perspective, then some interesting facts emerge. First, neither this woman nor Erickson used effortful thought to develop a solution. Instead, there was a surrendering of conscious effort to problem solve. Secondly, she was instructed to allow time for unconscious intelligence to identify her options by reviewing a lifetime of learning (implicit memories). Lastly, detailed instructions (prediction) were given for how to prepare for the solution's automatic arrival. Thus, a strong expectation was created for effortless, automatic behavior in the form of unconscious insight.

What seems to have occurred during the incubation period is that outside of awareness a question was both asked and answered, "By what means can I increase blood flow to my hands?" (implicit deliberation). At the appointed time, there was an unexplained reaction in her body that dramatically improved her circulation (implicit implementation). Because the woman's conscious reaction was fear and confusion, it seems probable that her conscious intelligence did not know about the question that had been asked or the insightful solution that was being implemented.

In competency-based therapies, the primary objective behind all psychotherapeutic endeavors is to stimulate the activation of unrecognized abilities for purposes determined by the will of the patient. Growth-oriented change is achieved by inviting the client to exercise choice and creative problem solving—often at unconscious levels. Whether it was the problem-solving step of defining the problem, identifying a solution, or implementing the solution, Erickson sought the involvement of the client's unconscious intelligence at all stages of the process. Often, this was achieved by creating *response expectancies* for unconscious insight, as we see demonstrated in this case.

9.1 Expectations Guide Automatic Behavior

As we look for a way to explain this approach to unconscious process work, it is helpful to turn to research conducted by Irving Kirsch and his *response expectancy theory*. This theory is based on the idea that automatic behavior is significantly influenced by people's expectations. As Kirsch (1985) puts it, response expectancies are expectancies of the occurrence of non-volitional responses, either as a function of behavior ("If I do X, then Y will automatically occur") or as a function of specific stimuli ("If I encounter X, then Y will automatically occur"). According to Kirsch, this is the mental process that produces placebo effects and hypnosis. The theory is supported by research showing that both subjective and physiological responses can be altered by changing people's expectancies. Another way of stating this is that expectancies trigger outcomes that do not seem to be under conscious control.

For example, Henry (1985) reported that people's preconceptions about hypnosis determined whether they reported time slowing down or speeding up, logical thought becoming easier or more difficult, the hypnotist's voice sounding closer or farther away, sounds being clearer or more muffled, and so forth. As an example of how these ideas have been tested, researchers Lynn, Rhue, and Weekes (1990) have shown that individuals informed that hypnotized people can resist suggestions succeed in resisting suggestions, whereas individuals told that hypnotized people cannot resist suggestions report a diminished ability to resist.

The same expectancy effects are found with placebos. As explained by Kirsch (1990), if you ask a person how they respond to alcohol, and they tell you that they become very sleepy, then when given a placebo drink (they believe is alcohol) the person becomes sleepy. If they expect to become humorous and more social with alcohol, then the placebo drink produces this response.

Interestingly, Kirsch is not the first to suspect that implicit expectations are important to healing. During the transition from magnetism to hypnosis, the French physician and neurologist Hippolyte Bernheim (1880) wrote that expectant attention turned inward on one's own experiences is the most likely explanation for healing that occurs during magnetism. What is special about Kirsch's response expectancy theory is that it not only unites the field of suggestive therapeutics (hypnosis and placebo therapies) but also connects the science of hypnosis to the well-established science of social learning theory.

While explaining response expectancy theory, Kirsch (1990, 10) equates response expectancies with self-fulfilling prophecy, stating, "When we expect to experience something strongly enough, we find ourselves actually experiencing it." Using experimental conditions, Kirsch and colleagues have shown that response expectancies can alter experiences of pain, nausea, tension, anxiety, depression, sexual arousal, and relaxation. What all of these have in common is that they are not amenable to change by means of conscious intention.

My reason for mentioning response expectancy in this chapter is because the activation of a problem-solving mindset at the level of unconscious intelligence is a special instance of automatic behavior. When we combine the use of expectancy effects with the use of an incubation period, the result is often profound and revelatory.

9.2 Incubated Cognition is Essential to Creative Insight

When an expert problem solver finds that his or her life is in danger, creative insights manifest (instantaneously) in action before there is time for thought. But for psychotherapy clientele, life-changing insights are more likely to emerge after a sequence of events. I can illustrate this progression in a brief case example.

My client was in her early thirties and suffering from severe anxiety and depression. As for appearances, her clothing was tight and provocative. As she joked about her "bad habit" of falling in love with married men, she leaned forward emphasizing her cleavage. After I asked for more details, she confessed to a sexual relationship with her boss. When I asked why this was a problem, she said he was married.

As the conversation continued, she slowly shifted her hips forward, causing her miniskirt to ride further up her thighs. Just as quickly as my eye was caught by the unexpected movement of her clothing, I turned my head, looking off to the right side of the room. Slipping into a state of reverie, I told her that I was thinking of someone who had a frightening experience. While staring into empty space, I told a story of a woman who had been careless and got herself into a situation that nearly resulted in gang rape and possible death. At the conclusion of the story, I slowly turned my head to meet with her eyes.

Her face had suddenly turned ashen. Her skirt was back down and as close to her knees as she could pull it. For a moment, she did not breathe. Then with a deep inhale she said,

> I was nearly raped after doing something really stupid. I had met a stranger on the train tracks and followed him to his house. I knew we were going there to have sex. But when I stepped inside, he bolted the

> door and looked at me with a sideways stare. That was when I filled with terror and realized that he planned to rape and kill me.

This story emotionally enriched her connection to me. She continued,

> I knew that I could not show my fear. Something told me to ask for a beer. Sitting down casually on his staircase, I told him that it would be more fun with alcohol. As soon as he walked into the kitchen, I jumped up, unlocked the door, and ran for my life.

I told her that this was excellent problem solving and that I was glad she was not harmed.

After sharing her story, she was in a state of acute psychological vulnerability, which was met with care and respect. I needed to demonstrate that she could tell me anything. As she shared more of her experiences, I helped her delineate those parts of her life that did not seem right (step 1: problem elaboration). She was horribly lonely and did not feel that she was of value to anyone else.

Next, I used my role as an expert to make a prediction, saying to her,

> You have done really good work during your therapy today. I believe you have impressive problem-solving abilities. When clients do this type of work during therapy, they often get surprising insights, most often it comes out of nowhere, as they are busy working on something else (step 2: create a response expectancy).

Two weeks later she returned to my office with an important insight (step 3). As she explained it to me, "By pursuing these men that are cheats … who do not really care about me … I am making myself unavailable for someone who might actually love me." The insight was powerful because it had taken root within her unconscious, and by the time it reached the surface of conscious awareness, it emerged with an explosion of emotion. She was proud of her insight, as was I. We then spent time discussing how this realization had important implications for many areas of her life (step 4: generalization). This moment in therapy was a major turning point.

The methodology I have just illustrated can be seen more clearly if we go back to the writings of Henri Poincaré (1854–1912), a mathematical genius who made the most significant advances in celestial mechanics since the time of Isaac Newton. As with many great thinkers, Poincaré was interested in the origins of his own astonishing creativity. He defined creativity as the identification of unsuspected relations among known facts, which is achieved in four cognitive phases: preparation, incubation, insight, and revision (Poincaré, 1908).

Preparation is the process during which the subject consciously studies the problem at hand (problem elaboration). During incubation, the subject's cognitive intelligence explores possibilities without conscious involvement—what Poincaré calls "the unconscious machine" (response expectancy). Next, there is a "sudden illumination" (insight). Lastly, for those who are scientifically trained, critical analysis follows the moment of inspiration as the new insights are evaluated and generalized to other areas of application (generalization).

Over one hundred years later, the effects of an incubation period continue to be studied. Now writers use the expression *unconscious incubated cognition* to indicate the actions of unconscious intelligence rather than something more random or coincidental, such as insight created by environmental primes. All those years ago, Poincaré (1908) made the same distinction when he wrote,

> it is not purely automatic; it is capable of discernment; it has tact and lightness of touch; it can divine. More than that, it can divine better than the conscious ego, since it succeeds where the latter fails.
>
> (57)

9.3 The Benefits of Unconscious Thought

The role of unconscious thought in producing insight has been studied closely by Ap Dijksterhuis of the University of Amsterdam and his colleagues. Dijksterhuis (2004) found that conscious thinking enables a person to follow precise rules using small amounts of information. However, unconscious processing permits the detection of meaningful patterns in an extremely large mass of information. This is the essence of unconscious thought theory (UTT), which was introduced by Dijksterhuis in 2004. In numerous studies he has shown that people make better decisions when they think about information unconsciously rather than consciously. The argument by Dijksterhuis and colleagues (2006) is that conscious thought is not capable of processing all the complex information that leads to the best decisions.

Once again, these are not new ideas. If we go back to America's first internationally recognized psychotherapeutic practitioner, Morton Prince (1854–1929) (1914), we find the following statement:

> [When asked a complex question] we consequently take the matter "under advisement," to use the conventional expression. We want time. And what we apparently ... do is to put the problem into our minds and leave it ... to incubate. ... we weigh, compare, and estimate the value of these different facts and arrive at a judgment. All happens as if subconscious processes have been at work, as if the problem has been going through a subconscious incubation, switching in this and switching in that set of facts, and presenting them to consciousness, the final selection of the deciding point of view being left to the latter. The subconscious garners from the store house of past experiences, those which have a bearing on the question and are required for its solution, brings them into consciousness, and then our logical conscious processes form the judgment.

> The degree to which subconscious processes in this way take part in informing judgments would vary according to the mental habits of the individual, the complexity of the problem, affectivity and conflicting character of the elements involved.
>
> (227–228)

Many now agree that an important aspect of productive incubation is that conscious attention needs to be diverted away from the problem. Scientists argue that successful performance on tasks that require creative recategorization (divergent thinking) is best accomplished by downregulation of the cognitive control regions. For example, one study found that when individuals were induced to allow their minds to wander, they showed an improvement of 40% compared to their baseline level of creative performance. This is achieved by simply saying "move the problem to the back of your mind" (Baird et al., 2012).

Neuroscientists, such as Jung-Beeman, have speculated that during the *preparatory phase* of insight-oriented problem solving, the instinctual tendency to close one's eyes and push aside all linguistic thought has the functional advantage of allowing the cortex to be free of distraction. This allows neural activity to shift to the more remote associations that are processed in the right hemisphere—the brain region that provides the insight. Jung-Beeman argues that a *relaxation phase* is crucial to insight, and that is why so many insights happen while taking a warm shower or strolling through the woods (Lehrer, 2012). This might also help explain why practitioners of hypnosis continue to embrace the clinical tradition of having problem solvers close their eyes, cease effortful conscious thought, and spend 20 to 40 minutes in a relaxed state. As insight researcher John Kounios puts it, "If you want to encourage insights, then you've got to also encourage people to relax" (Lehrer, 2008, 40).

In addition to conscious surrender and relaxation, a third crucial element in preparation for insight is time. When tested, longer unconscious thought leads to better decisions than brief unconscious thought (Dijksterhuis, 2004). Using meta-analysis, Sio and Ormerod (2009) found that longer preparation periods gave a greater incubation effect, whereas filling an incubation period with high cognitive demand tasks produced a smaller incubation effect. Also, low cognitive demand tasks (mind wandering) yielded a stronger incubation effect than rest did during an incubation period when solving insight problems. Most importantly, they found that incubation works best for problems that require creative solutions (divergent thinking).

The general implication of these findings is that postponing a complex decision for as long as possible is advantageous, even if one does not consciously think about it during this period. When faced with complex demands, people who understand this strategy will assert themselves, saying, "Let me get back with you once I have an answer."

In the clinical context, incubated cognition might be employed for a period of minutes, days, weeks, or even years. This is achieved by establishing response expectancies using expert opinion or prediction.

For example, a client asked me yesterday, "How will I know if I should marry this woman or break up with her and look for someone different?" I include this as an example because many therapists have been asked these types of questions. The typical guidance we receive from mainstream psychotherapy is: do not attempt to make that decision for them! If you do, then you are responsible for outcomes you cannot control. I have sad stories I could tell about people who lost marriages after being advised by a therapist to divorce (with both living in isolation until their death) and more than one woman who lost her life after being told that she must pack her bags and leave an abusive relationship (the violent partner decided not to allow it). This rule helps distinguish trained professionals from well-intentioned friends, who never hesitate to give advice.

Even professional opinions can be harmful if it causes the client to circumvent his or her own self-understanding and implicit knowledge. But what do we do to help clients gain the insight they are hoping to achieve? Returning to the client seeking marriage advice, he asked this question because he was 38 years old and eager to start a family. He had already broken up with his girlfriend once before because he felt she was overly controlling, did not take good care of her body, and did not like any of his friends or the types of things he enjoyed doing, such as hiking or camping. Before attempting to set any response expectancies, I collected more information, asking if he was currently living with her. I learned that his plan was to ask her to move in with him soon. Next, I wanted to know whether he would give the relationship a third try if he did break up again. He insisted that he was committed to one of two options: either get married or break up and meet someone new. So, I asked, "What is the absolute longest amount of time that you are willing to wait until you get an answer to your question?" He said, six months—starting after they move in together. With these facts in mind, I set up an insight response expectancy, saying,

> Six months is plenty of time for your unconscious mind to determine what type of wife she would be and whether she is a good fit for you. This is not something you will be able to discern consciously. There are too many variables, and there are future expectations for what married life should be, which she may not tell you. But the unconscious picks up on these things. The way you will know is by the feeling in your heart or in your gut. It will be a strong, visceral feeling. You may not be able to explain why, but one day you will clearly know what you must do. When that day comes, I strongly encourage you to act on what your body is telling you to do. It will be the wisest choice you could possibly make.

This prediction is open-ended but not without structure. While he could have his insight as soon as he was ready, I set a deadline that was as remote as he was willing to accept (six months). This is a reasonable incubation period to discern with whom to spend the rest of your life. Remember, the longer the incubation period, the better the final decision.

For those clients who feel less able to state how long they can wait for an answer, I set a pseudo time point, saying, "Your unconscious will take just as long as it needs to produce the right solution. When the answer comes, you may not know how you know, but you can trust that for you this is the right solution." If a client asks me how I can be so certain, I describe the research on incubated cognition and share with them as many empirically derived facts or case examples as they care to hear. However, whenever possible, it is best to get the client to forecast how long he or she will need to arrive at a confident decision.

9.4 The Architect versus the Archaeologist

In agreement with Schopenhauer, William James believed that unconscious processes are a vital resource for problem solving and the foundation upon which we construct our conscious intention. James viewed the unconscious mind as the organizing center of personality (James, 1902, 206). Thus, when comparing it to the conscious mind, James stated that the unconscious mind is "far wiser than and superior to that of normal, waking, rational awareness" (Taylor, 1982, 91). At a later date James (1916) explained,

> It is but a small part of our experience in life that we are ever able articulately to recall. And yet the whole of it has had its influence in shaping the character and defining our tendencies to judge and act. (142)

The point that James makes has been elaborated by Dijksterhuis and Nordgren (2016) in terms of the *capacity principle*: unconscious thought has a much higher processing capacity than conscious thought. Thus, conscious thought by necessity often considers only a subset of the relevant information. With access to a larger pool of information, unconscious intelligence is better able to weigh the relative importance of various variables (*weighting principle*).

These authors argue that conscious thought often leads to suboptimal weighting because it leads people to put disproportionate weight on attributes that are accessible, plausible, and easy to verbalize (stereotypes). These ill-conceived conclusions then become a distraction to unconscious processes, like a runner who jumps the gun and throws the race. As Dijksterhuis and Nordgren (2016) point out, it is hard to avoid "jumping to conclusions" when using conscious thought. It may feel as if one is processing information with the goal of making an informed decision, however, unknowingly, one is processing information with the goal of confirming an expectancy.

Conversely, Dijksterhuis and colleagues have found that some problems are better handled by conscious intelligence. For example, conscious thinking enables a person to follow precise rules using small amounts of information. In a therapy setting, if a woman is in need of an order of protection, then it is best to help her consciously consider the steps that must be taken and the order in which they are to be implemented. For this type of intellectual task, we might offer the individual a pen and paper to take notes. These notes then serve as a prime that helps reengage *conscious* deliberation.

In contrast, incubated cognition enables a person to detect critical patterns in a mass of information. This is the type of intelligence that is needed when it is important to "see the big picture." In a therapy setting, if a woman was trying to decide whether to marry one person or another, then this decision would be best processed outside of conscious awareness. If she tried to depend entirely on her conscious intelligence, she might fail to take into account critical information stored outside of conscious awareness.

In other words, decisions about orderly, rule-governed issues are best processed in conscious thought, whereas *decisions about complex or chaotic situations require unconscious process work*. For example, research by Tilmann Betsch and colleagues (2001) demonstrates that unconscious thought can detect patterns in numbers and produce rough estimates on the basis of these details (inductive logic) but does not engage in arithmetic, which is precise and rule governed. Thus, unconscious intelligence can deal with numbers to some extent, but not by doing arithmetic. Similarly, Kahneman (2011) argued that unconscious thought is not capable of probabilistic reasoning (deductive logic).

Dijksterhuis helps us understand these differences by comparing conscious thought to the work of an architect—it solves problems using a single set of blueprints. In contrast, unconscious thought is more like an archaeologist—it solves problems by piecing together obscure details. This is the same difference we find in deductive reasoning versus inductive reasoning. Deductive logic uses a single law or principle to explain many different things (schematic processing). It is essentially intellectual stereotyping, which in academia has been criticized as *scientific reductionism*.

In contrast, *inductive logic* expansively seeks out details, just as Sherlock Holmes would intuitively piece together clues to solve a crime (yes, sadly, Holmes was misleading Watson each time he called it deduction). Recall all that we have learned about unconscious perception and its *enormous* capacity and sensitivity (subliminal perception). It is not difficult to see why inductive reasoning is intuitive—conducted mostly outside of conscious awareness. Therefore, people sometimes talk about the "art of doing psychotherapy." It is another way of saying: this person was able to think outside of the box (aschematic processing) by relying on implicit cognition to conduct inductive analysis and produce an outcome that cannot be fully accounted for by one's conscious intelligence.

This leads us back to Poincaré's stage theory, or what Dijksterhuis and Nordgren (2016) call the "best of both worlds" hypothesis: Complex decisions are best when the information is encoded thoroughly and consciously (*preparation*), and the later thought process is delegated to the unconscious (*incubation*). Applying this principle to psychotherapy, when a client is struggling with an overwhelming problem, the first step is to help him or her consciously acquire as much relevant information as possible prior to incubated cognition.

Thus, when a client is seeking insight into a complex problem, my version of talk therapy is mostly me asking questions about the details of the problem or me sharing psychological data, as if I were conducting a lecture in social psychology. I am not offering an opinion on what the client should do but rather equipping the client with concepts that later act as tools for unconscious deliberation. During this stage, I want the client to ask me questions or disagree with my comments so that the information can be elaborated and thoroughly processed.

The next step is the weighting and evaluation of information needed to arrive at a judgment. This is when it is helpful to create a response expectancy that the solution to the problem is best left to unconscious intelligence. For example, I might say,

> Your unconscious will continue to work on this problem, even as you sleep and dream of different potential realities. There is no need to consciously think about it. It is best to focus on other relaxing tasks. But if you suddenly wake up in the middle of the night after a profound dream, or if you suddenly see something that causes a powerful emotional response, know that this is your unconscious seeking to reveal its solution.

9.5 Estimating the Length of an Incubation Period

In a laboratory experiment by Dijksterhuis and van Olden (2006), students were asked to choose an art poster to take home. Weeks later they were more satisfied with their choice if they were distracted before making their decision compared to those who could engage in conscious deliberation. Numerous studies such as this have led Dijksterhuis to conclude that unconscious cognition is particularly good at forecasting emotional responses, especially when it comes to highly complex events.

Studies such as these become highly relevant to psychotherapy if we think of the space between sessions as a potential incubation period. Each new session holds the possibility of intense emotionality as implicit self-knowledge or unconscious knowledge about others is revealed to conscious awareness. The question is: How long of an incubation period does the client need so that he or she is fully prepared for whatever might need to take place during therapy?

Rather than adhering to a routine schedule, I invite my clients to estimate the best length of time between sessions. I accomplish this by asking, "When does it feel like you should come back? When will you be emotionally ready? What is the first thing that pops into your head?" On the surface, these questions just sound polite. If we look more closely, we can see that they set up a response expectancy: "When you do return, a significant emotional response will occur." I am not asking the client to consciously consider what they should discuss during the next appointment, but the response expectancy will automatically activate incubated cognition.

Sometimes a client will say during a therapy session, "I do not think I am ready to know." We might be talking about a girlfriend (who could be cheating), a spouse (who could die during surgery), or a memory from childhood (that could be very disturbing). Regardless of the topic, my response is, "How long do you think you will need?" The person's answer helps initiate an incubation period during which the unconscious seeks to answer a very important question—how will I cope with this new knowledge when it becomes conscious? I learned this strategy from Erickson, who was careful to establish timeframes for new understandings that were derived entirely from the client's own emotional forecasting.

Of course, it is also possible for incubated cognition to occur during a session. If I am discussing a highly emotional topic with a client, I will slow down my speech so that it is possible for the client to become lost in revery as I speak. When there are long gaps between sentences during a very inwardly absorbing topic, clients can become so involved in processing that they are not consciously aware of being in a conversation with someone else. As their eyes look off into some space beside them, I just wait. When the person looks back towards my face, I know that the incubation period has ended. Fifteen minutes is about the longest I have had to wait for someone to re-engage in the conversation. More often, it is only a minute or two. On these occasions I do not ask what the person was thinking because that interferes with the unconscious nature of the self-exploration.

As Dijksterhuis has shown experimentally, conscious deliberative reasoning can dampen the quality of self-knowledge. In studies when people were asked to deliberate on their preferences, it was found that they were less consistent than those who made non-deliberative judgments. We have been taught to expect more reliable information from careful, deliberative thought. But when the subject of observation is the emotional self (or other extremely complex systems), conscious deliberation tends to cloud perception. As Nordgren and Dijksterhuis (2009, 45) put it, "our judgmental apparatus is far from flawless. And ironically, it gets worse when we deliberate." If we wish for our clients to be at their intellectual best during psychotherapy, then we must make certain that we match the task to the corresponding intelligence. The greater the mass of variables that must be weighed, the more creative the solution must be, or the more emotionally overwhelming the subject matter, the better it is to use incubated cognition without conscious involvement.

9.6 Forced Mental Effort can Interfere with Unconscious Productivity

The sometimes paradoxical effect of conscious intention was of great interest to Fyodor Dostoevsky (1863, 49), who described his thought experiment, "Try to pose for yourself this task: not to think of a polar bear, and you will see that the cursed thing will come to mind every minute." This effect is now known as ironic rebound.

Also curious about the limitations of conscious intention, Charles Darwin (1809–1882) conducted a psychophysiological experiment. After gathering a small group of men interested in taking a wager, Darwin asked about their reactions to snuff. Each man insisted that the substance made him sneeze. Their collective belief was that the sneezing was uncontrollable and could not be prevented by force of will. In response to the men, Darwin wagered the opposite. He offered to pay a small sum of money to anyone who was able to sneeze in response to a pinch of snuff. Each took their pinch, but no matter how hard they tried, none could sneeze. Several of the men's eyes watered, so they knew it was not a trick. The snuff was real enough, but not a single one of them could sneeze. This was the outcome Darwin had predicted. Later, Darwin (1872) commented, "The conscious wish to perform a reflex action sometimes stops or interrupts its performance" (42). Prior to the invention of depth psychology, Darwin had recognized that effortful conscious attention can interfere with unconscious activity.

This phenomenon has been studied extensively by Harvard psychologist Daniel Wegner within the frame of ironic process theory. As Wegner (2002) explains, many of our most important goals, when pursued consciously, result not just in failure but in the ironic opposite of that goal. In other words, when consciously trying to be happy, we are likely to become depressed, or distracted when we force ourselves to concentrate, or wide awake when we try to make ourselves sleep, and as noted by Dostoevsky, when trying to forget, we remember the object all the more clearly.

Ironic effects are not confined to physical reflexes, emotions, imagery, and autonomic activity (trying to fall asleep), they also extend to the realm of thought and perception. In research, subjects who were instructed to be fair and unprejudiced became more prejudiced. Even more insidious is the effect known as "moral licensing." When a person is prompted to make a public positive moral self-evaluation, subsequent behavior will move in the opposite direction.

For example, Monin and Miller (2001) found that those who establish that they are not prejudiced are more likely to exhibit prejudice behaviors in follow up exercises. Similarly, shoppers who make a conscious effort to buy at least one environmentally responsible product are more likely to subsequently purchase self-indulgent products (Khan and Dhar 2006). Imagine the trouble that might result when the more we assert ourselves in one direction, the further we secretly travel down the opposite path.

It is little wonder that people sometimes feel that they have lost control over their lives. Think of the unfortunate alcoholic who publicly declares that he will never drink again! Or the husband who assures his wife that he would never cheat on her and then offers up an example of his chastity (this is the same as buying one environmentally responsible product). This helps explain the superstitious fear of "jinxing" one's self. The problems that come with declaring a conscious intention are both comical and tragic. Rather than knocking on wood or throwing salt over our shoulder, *we need to avoid relying on conscious intention to implement behaviors that are automatic in nature.* When we need to declare our intentions, it should be done with a spirit of humility.

"Let go and let God," is a slogan that people in twelve-step recovery groups often quote. It is meant to convey the importance of surrender and of no longer seeking to consciously control one's problem-solving efforts. If we stop to consider how this strategy could help shield a person from harmful rebound effects and moral licensing while simultaneously creating positive response expectancy effects, then it is easy to see why the strategy has been so successful with those who are trying to solve massively complex life problems.

With problems such as alcoholism, we are dealing with behaviors that people wish to eliminate. However, the more they try to force themselves to not do this thing or not feel a certain way, the less access they have to the problem-solving capabilities of unconscious intelligence. I mention the slogan from AA because it is a good example of an implementation intention (action plan) designed to achieve problem-solving activity outside of conscious awareness. As we would expect, research by Gollwitzer and colleagues (2002) found that implementation intentions insulate an individual's goals from ironic rebound effects by minimizing the use of effortful conscious control.

The exact same dynamic is achieved in psychotherapy by telling the person,

> Your brain is made to solve problems without you thinking about it. But there are certain things that will help your unconscious process better. It may be hiking in the hills, visiting with close friends, or praying in a church. Whatever the activity is, you will feel that you are getting closer to something important without having to think about it. Tell me, what activity does your gut tell you that you should do while your unconscious is busy working on a solution?

With this exchange there is the creation of response expectancies as well as implementation intention and a virtual boundary that solidifies commitment. This all fits with the goal of unconscious process work, which is to encourage and validate people as they move in the direction of trusting their own innate capabilities while utilizing a lifetime of unconscious learnings and realizing a shared expectation for progress and creative problem solving.

As with each technique described in this book, incubated cognition is a growth-oriented means of problem solving that points the client in the direction of his or her own self-efficacy. The experience of competency is not as closely connected to deliberate behavior as it is to automatic behavior. For example, when a winning athlete is "in the zone" he or she pushes past old barriers while hardly thinking. The problem solving feels automatic and effortless. As Stokes (2007, 95) puts it, "Incubated processing is important to creativity *because* it is important to how we learn, practice, and engage with novel tasks, skills, and information—how we are capable of cognitive novelty." Thus, unconscious incubated cognition is one of those essential skills that can be learned in psychotherapy and then applied to a lifetime of everyday problem solving.

Chapter 9 Key Points

- Meaningful insight involves unconscious problem solving (incubated cognition).
- Incubated cognition is more likely to engage if we expect it to occur.
- Conscious thought is poorly suited for weighing the complex variables in major life decisions.
- Decisions about orderly, rule-governed issues are best processed in conscious thought, whereas decisions about chaotic situations require unconscious processing.
- The greater the mass of variables that must be weighed, the more creative the solution must be, or the more emotionally overwhelming the subject matter, the better it is to use incubated cognition without conscious involvement.
- Overdependence on conscious intention sets people up for ironic behavior.

References

Baird, Benjamin, Jonathan Smallwood, Michael D. Mrazek, Julia W. Y. Kam, Michael S. Franklin, and Jonathan W. Schooler. 2012. "Inspired by Distraction: Mind Wandering Facilitates Creative Incubation." *Psychological Science* 23 (10): 1117–1122. doi:10.1177/0956797612446024.

Bernheim, Hippolyte. (1880) 2006. *Suggestive Therapeutics: A Treatise On The Nature And Uses Of Hypnotism*. Translated by Christian A. Herter. Whitefish, MT: Kessinger Publishing, LLC.

Betsch, Tilmann, Henning Plessner, Christiane Schwieren, and Robert Gütig. 2001. "I like It But I Don't Know Why: A Value-Account Approach to Implicit Attitude Formation." *Personality and Social Psychology Bulletin* 27 (2): 242–253. doi:10.1177/0146167201272009.

Bowden, Edward M., Mark Jung-Beeman, Jessica Fleck, and John Kounios. 2005. "New Approaches to Demystifying Insight." *Trends in Cognitive Sciences* 9 (7): 322–328. doi:10.1016/j.tics.2005.05.012.

Darwin, Charles. 1872. *The Expression of Emotion in Animals and Man*. London: Methuen.

Dijksterhuis, Ap. 2004. "Think Different: The Merits of Unconscious Thought in Preference Development and Decision Making." *Journal of Personality and Social Psychology* 87 (5): 586–598. doi:10.1037/0022-3514.87.5.586.

Dijksterhuis, Ap, Maarten W. Bos, Loran F. Nordgren, and Rick B. van Baaren. 2006. "On Making the Right Choice: The Deliberation-Without-Attention Effect." *Science* 311 (5763): 1005–1007. doi:10.1126/science.1121629.

Dijksterhuis, Ap, and Teun Meurs. 2006. "Where Creativity Resides: The Generative Power of Unconscious Thought." *Conscious Cognition* 15 (1): 135–146. doi:10.1016/j.concog.2005.04.007.

Dijksterhuis, Ap, and Loran F. Nordgren. 2016. "A Theory of Unconscious Thought:" *Perspectives on Psychological Science* 1 (2): 95–109. doi:10.1111/j.1745-6916.2006.00007.x.

Dijksterhuis, Ap, and Zeger van Olden. 2006. "On the Benefits of Thinking Unconsciously: Unconscious Thought Can Increase Post-Choice Satisfaction." *Journal of Experimental Social Psychology* 42 (5): 627–631. doi:10.1016/j.jesp.2005.10.008.

Dostoevsky, Fyodor. (1863) 1997. *Winter Notes on Summer Impressions.* Translated by David Patterson. Evanston, IL: Northwestern University Press.

Erickson, Milton H. 1960. *A Lecture by Milton H. Erickson: Chicago, June 10, 1960.* (Audio Recording No. CD/EMH.60.3.21). CD. Phoenix, AZ: The Milton H. Erickson Foundation Archives.

Freud, Sigmund. (1900) 1966. "The Interpretation Of Dreams." In *The Basic Writings of Sigmund Freud*, translated and edited by A. A. Brill, 181–468. New York: Random House.

Gollwitzer, P. M., R. Trotschel, and M. Sumner. 2002. "Mental Control via Implementation Intentions Is Void of Rebound Effects." Unpublished Manuscript, University of Konstanz.

Henry, David C. 1985. *Subjects' Expectancies and Subjective Experience of Hypnosis.* PhD dissertation. University of Connecticut.

James, William. (1902) 1985. *The Varieties of Religious Experience.* Boston, MA: Harvard University Press.

James, William. 1916. *Talks To Teachers On Psychology; And To Students On Some Of Life's Ideals.* New York: Henry Holt. Project Gutenberg. http://www.gutenberg.org/ebooks/16287.

Kahneman, Daniel. 2011. *Thinking, Fast and Slow.* New York: Farrar, Straus and Giroux.

Khan, Uzma, and Ravi Dhar. 2006. "Licensing Effect in Consumer Choice." *Journal of Marketing Research* 43 (2): 259–266. doi:10.1509/jmkr.43.2.259.

Kirsch, Irving. 1985. "Response Expectancy as a Determinant of Experience and Behavior." *American Psychologist* 40 (11): 1189–1202.

Kirsch, Irving. 1990. *Changing Expectations: A Key to Effective Psychotherapy.* Belmont, CA: Thomson Brooks/Cole Publishing Co.

Lehrer, Jonah. 2008. "The Eureka Hunt." *The New Yorker*, July 28. https://www.newyorker.com/magazine/2008/07/28/the-eureka-hunt.

Lehrer, Jonah. 2012. *Imagine: How Creativity Works.* 1st edition. New York: Houghton Mifflin.

Lynn, Steven J., Judith W. Rhue, and John R. Weekes. 1990. "Hypnotic Involuntariness: A Social Cognitive Analysis." *Psychological Review* 97 (2): 169–184. doi:10.1037/0033-295X.97.2.169.

McLuhan, Marshall. 1962. *The Gutenberg Galaxy: The Making of Typographic Man.* Toronto: University of Toronto Press.

Monin, Benoit, and Dale T. Miller. 2001. "Moral Credentials and the Expression of Prejudice." *Journal of Personality and Social Psychology* 81 (1): 33–43. doi:10.1037/0022-3514.81.1.33.

Neubauer, Peter B. 1979. "The Role of Insight in Psychoanalysis." *Journal of the American Psychoanalytic Association* 27 (Suppl.): 29–40.

Nordgren, Loran F., and Ap Dijksterhuis. 2009. "The Devil Is in the Deliberation: Thinking Too Much Reduces Preference Consistency." *Journal of Consumer Research* 36 (1): 39–46. doi:10.1086/596306.

Poincaré, Henri. (1908) 1914. *Science and Method*. Translated by Francis Maitland. London: Thomas Nelson and Sons.

Prince, Morton. (1914) 1921. *The Unconscious: The Fundamentals of Human Personality Normal and Abnormal*. New York: Macmillan.

Sio, Ut Na, and Thomas C. Ormerod. 2009. "Does Incubation Enhance Problem Solving?: A Meta-Analytic Review." *Psychological Bulletin* 135 (1): 94–120. doi:10.1037/a0014212.

Stokes, Dustin. 2007. "Incubated Cognition and Creativity." *Journal of Consciousness Studies* 14 (3): 83–100.

Taylor, Eugene. 1982. *William James on Exceptional Mental States: The 1896 Lowell Lectures*. New York: Scribner.

10 Unconscious Process Work: A Growth Mindset

To better digest this large body of ideas, recall that Chapter 1 frames unconscious process work as a strategic problem-solving methodology. This methodology places unconscious abilities in the lead position during tandem work with conscious intelligence. Chapter 2 makes the argument that unconscious processes have access to greater information than conscious knowledge. Chapter 3 argues for the existence of an unconscious intelligence that is capable of setting goals, monitoring progress, and exercising non-volitional will. Chapter 4 considers the importance of cross-talk between conscious and unconscious intelligences so that there is less division and conflict within the mind. Then, Chapter 5 argues that there is a special vocabulary better suited to an unconscious intelligence, which should be used to communicate ideas that are more advanced and structurally complex than what can be handled by conscious thought.

In the second half of the book, we get into more detailed information on how to therapeutically engage unconscious processes. Starting with Chapter 6, the need to engage unconscious problem solving to achieve an explicit goal is addressed by making highly motivating predictions. In Chapter 7, the need to exercise choice over the effect of one's life experiences (self-determination) is addressed through imaginative involvement and creativity. In Chapter 8, the need to activate goal-oriented behavior, without requiring conscious attention for implementation, is addressed through a structured goal-setting and planning process. Then, Chapter 9 addresses the need for unconscious deliberation and divergent problem solving by creating the expectation that this will occur during an incubation period. The objective for Chapter 10 is to embed all this clinical knowledge more deeply in a part of the mind that does not easily forget. I would explain how this will be engineered, but that would prematurely silence unconscious processes.

10.1 Motivation

Using effortless imagination, picture yourself sitting in your office with a couple sitting across from you. Their marriage is in crisis, and the woman is clearly in a great deal of pain. The man is contrite. He says he feels bad about cheating on his wife, yet he remains emotionally closed off.

DOI: 10.4324/9781003127208-10

Based on this presentation, you predict that it is the wife who will be most willing to share information. You invite her to provide a narrative of what has occurred. From her story you learn that the husband repeatedly lied about how many women he sought attention from (mostly by phone) and how much physical contact he had with them. At times he has been hostile towards the wife, yelling at her and blaming her personality and physique for his marital infidelity. When he is not traveling for work, he spends most of the day sleeping late and isolating himself from his wife and children. The wife reports that two days ago she became so angry that she was ready to file for divorce. But now she has decided to give the marriage a second chance.

What is your response? Who would you address first, and how would you initiate unconscious process work? What is the first thing that pops into your mind? Pause for a moment to see what ideas come to you.

As with most problems brought into the therapy office, at first this marriage seems like a lost cause. But as you imagine your response, begin by imaging a successful ending. You need to be able to envision a positive future so that you are properly motivated (promotion motivation). My experience has been that the only instance when a well-trained therapist can no longer help troubled individuals is when they are not really seeking help in the first place.

Observing that the man was the one exercising the most power in the relationship, I felt that he was in the best position to make things right. My question to him was, "Did you intend to treat your wife this way? Did you plan to become an abusive husband?"

He was deeply ashamed of his actions. The harshness of my question reflected his current self-understanding. He did not become defensive, presumably because he felt my comments were accurate. Instead, he told me he did not want to be this type of person. But he also insisted that he did not understand why he was doing these things.

As a psychologist, I am willing to render my expert opinion on why certain behaviors are occurring, but not until I have first verified my hunches with at least three pieces of evidence. So, I asked him, "When you are alone in a hotel room sending text messages to other women, is there alcohol involved?" He answers, "Yes." So, I asked, "When you get into hostile emotional states and yell at your wife, have you been drinking earlier in the day?" He answers, "Yes." So, I ask, "When you stay in bed, not getting up with the family, is your head hurting? Do you feel hungover?" He answers, "Yes." After this, I was ready to make my predictions.

I sized up the situation this way, "Each time you have cheated on your wife, you have been drinking. Each time you verbally assault your wife, you have been drinking. Alcohol seems to be controlling you in undesirable ways." Because he had no arguments with my logic, I continued with my predictions, "If you quit drinking, you may be able to save your marriage. You certainly will have better control of your behavior."

After I got him to answer some more questions about his drinking history, his wife was shocked. He had hidden most of his drinking. His wife had mistakenly attributed his change in personality to a back injury, which coincided with when he started drinking heavily.

Next, I made a second prediction,

> You may think that you can just decide to quit drinking and that will be it. Because most people who are alcoholics do not realize it at first. But if you go back to drinking and risk losing your family, then you will have to admit that you are an alcoholic.

His wife asked me what she should do if he starts drinking again. I told her that she should demand he leave the house and find himself a room to rent.

To his credit, the husband almost achieved two weeks without alcohol. But then he ended up in a medical hospital for two days and a psychiatric hospital for four nights after overdosing on antidepressant medication, alcohol, and Benadryl. He came very close to dying.

In the couple's next session, I learned that he had not been planning the suicide attempt. Rather, it was an impulsive act that developed during a state of intoxication. Once again, I focused his attention on the prominence of alcohol in all his troubles, including the affair. This time he openly admitted that alcohol had been destroying his marriage and his life. With the help of an individual therapist for him (I only conducted couples counseling) and daily AA meetings, he made it four weeks with no alcohol.

During this time, he was a transformed person. He was considerate, playful, and grateful to his wife. He helped take care of household chores and was more involved with the children. Then he got his hands on a bottle of vodka. Immediately, he began to belittle his wife, lie to her about having had any alcohol, and send text messages to the woman he had been physically involved with.

It was clear what his explicit goal needed to be—no more alcohol ever again. But what prediction could be used to organize unconscious planning around this objective?

Stop for a little while and see what ideas pop into your mind.

During the session, the husband was quiet. It was his wife that was doing most of the talking. She asked me why he did this. I asked him if he could explain. He said he could not find an explanation other than to say he is an alcoholic. By making this confession, he crossed a virtual boundary. This both strengthened his commitment to change and the power of my predictions.

Next, I asked how he felt after going back to drinking. He replied, "Horrible!" It was clear from his words and demeanor that he felt terrible remorse. I asked if he had planned to do this after the last time we talked, and he insisted he had not. Clearly, his conscious intentions were not going to save him from this problem.

So, I shifted causal attributions to his unconscious thought processes by saying, "Almost all alcoholics relapse. Often, there is a question that the unconscious mind needs answered, 'Do I really want to quit?' So, there is one last test." Then, I made two crucial predictions. The first was designed to produce hope, "For those who feel horrible afterwards and experience deep remorse, it is often the last time they drink." I then followed that happy outcome with a severe contrast, "For others, they must feel even worse, so they keep drinking until their wife divorces them. Or, they attempt suicide yet again, and then finally they decide 'never again.'" The two predictions represented a fork in the road with both paths leading in the same direction—stop drinking.

Six months later, at the time of this writing, he has remained sober. He wakes every morning at 5:00 a.m. to exercise and do his AA meditations. He has lost 25 pounds and no longer requires antidepressant medication. His wife states that she is pleased and proud of her husband. She credits him with inspiring her to take better care of herself, and as a result she has lost weight as well.

Although this anecdotal account does not prove anything about the efficacy of the techniques that were employed, it does illustrate the importance of not giving up on clients just because their preexistent problem-solving resources have not been sufficient for the challenges they face. If at some point in the future this client relapses, which is probable, I will continue to engage his conscious and unconscious resources in service of growth-oriented problem-solving.

When seeking to use clinical prediction in your own practice, keep in mind that *you are not attempting to foresee the future, but rather to enable it.* Prediction implicitly activates fantasy and imagination as well as prefactual information. These images of the future then function as a highly motivating prime that locks into unconscious working memory (due to the heightened state of anticipation). While personal power is most productive when checked by responsibility, a positive prediction helps provide the energy and hope needed to move forward. As a rule, use predictions as prescriptions (only when needed), leaving plenty of space for self-determination, unexpected developments, and self-discovery.

10.2 Creativity and Choice

Now imagine a different couple sitting in front of you. The wife has her arms crossed and her face is contorted in an angry scowl. Sitting at her side is her husband, who has sunk into the couch, and his crumpled face shows signs of exhaustion and failure.

Picture this couple in your office, and the woman dominates the conversation, repeatedly making the point that her husband has brought her nothing but shame and disappointment. Her primary complaint is that he does not show that he loves her. Defensively, the husband counters, "But I do try, really hard. But nothing I do is ever good enough."

To make her point, she orders her husband to tell you, the therapist, what he bought her for Christmas. The man starts to plead,

> That was just a place holder! I told you, I had been walking around the mall for hours. None of the gifts were good enough. I just bought that as a placeholder, with a note in the box saying we would go out together to buy you a real Christmas gift.

The woman then turns to you with contempt in her voice, "He bought me a bottle of Curél hand lotion! Tell me, what kind of husband buys his wife hand lotion for Christmas?!" Before you have time to answer, she turns back on her husband, "You humiliated me in front of my family! I had to go to the bedroom because I could not stop crying. A loving husband would never do this to his wife!"

Now they turn their attention to you, waiting for you to somehow make things better. If you are hoping for their conscious intelligence to be able to solve this problem, as I was, then you will ask the wrong question, as I did.

Looking her in the eyes, I asked, "Have you told him what types of things he can do so that you feel loved?" This only made her feel more exasperated—I suppose I now seemed as dumb as her husband.

Rolling her eyes, she explained, "If you are having to tell someone what to do so that they can seem loving, it is no longer proof that they actually love you." I sought clarification, "So he has to figure out for himself what he has to do to make you feel that he sincerely loves you." Her reply, "Yes."

While trying to buy time for my unconscious intelligence to devise a strategy, I told her my frank opinion, which was that her husband would continue to fail at this task, just as he had in the past. Her reply was, "Then this marriage will not last."

Now imagine looking over at the man. He is not angry. He has a look of sadness on his face. He does not want to lose his marriage to divorce. The use of reason and logic are off the table.

What are you going to do to help introduce the opportunity for collaborative problem solving? Better yet, how do you create an experience in the office that will automatically trigger a strong attachment response? Unless she drops her defenses, she will not be able to see that her husband loves her deeply.

If you want to get the most from this exercise, stop to imagine at least three or four possibilities before reading further. Allow yourself to free associate.

Knowing that her confidence in me had dissolved, I attempted to better acknowledge her subjective reality by saying, "I see a lot of pain in your eyes. I think you have been hurt deeply and that this pain is interfering with your marriage." She nods in agreement and flashes a glance at her husband. He looks worried, as if I have now turned on him. But I was not thinking of her husband.

Leaning in, I told her, "This pain was there before your marriage. How old were you when it first happened?" She asked me what I meant. I clarified, "When you first felt this pain, were you a child or a teenager?" As if her awareness was no longer completely oriented to the present moment, she replied, "A teenager … I was sixteen." She then became watery eyed and looked frightened. She sunk into the couch. All her aggression suddenly vanished.

Her husband spoke up for her, "She was raped at that age. She does not like to talk about it."

I asked her if this was true, and she nodded yes. I told her I was sorry that it had happened and that she did not deserve to have someone do that to her. Using an apologetic tone, I explained to her, "I do not want to bring up something that is uncomfortable for you. But I am afraid this bad experience is affecting your marriage. I think we need to address your past for your marriage to have a future."[1]

I now had a hunch about what might be helpful. But I wanted to collect some evidence before acting on my hunch, so I asked her, "When you fell in love with your husband, did you feel safe with him? Is that part of the reason you wanted to marry him?" She said that I was correct. I asked a second question, "If you were in danger, would he hesitate to protect you?" She shook her head no. To increase the emotional impact, I asked, "Would he be willing to lay down his life, if he had to, in order to protect you?" She turned to look at her husband. He asserted himself, "I absolutely would." I said, "Good."

Then I told the wife that if she felt I was a capable therapist, and if she felt she could trust me, then I would need her to leave the couch and sit in the hypnosis chair. After she complied, I told her,

> I could conduct hypnosis with you and go back in time to change your emotional experience about the trauma. And, it would probably help a little. However, if your husband does the hypnosis, it will be much more effective for you.
>
> I then asked, "Are you willing to allow your husband to help you?" She nodded yes.

The husband was rightfully concerned that he might not be able to do hypnosis. I assured him that I would tell him exactly what to say and do.

His first instructions were to ask his wife to tell him all the details that she could remember from the sexual assault. Her eyes were closed, and she cried as she described being chased through a park late at night, desperately looking for someone to rescue her. After enough details were collected, I had him start to guide her through the memory, reconstructing it just as she had described the event.

Then, when it came to the crucial moment, just as the predator was about to grab her, I had him introduce himself into the scene. I told him to describe to her what he was prepared to do to that criminal in order to keep her safe. I then instructed him on what words to say so that she could feel her personal power once again. Up until this moment, her body had been trembling.

After she breathed deeply and became still, I suggested that he touch his wife on the shoulder so that she could feel that he was *really* there for her—

that he truly loved her. With her eyes still closed, she reached up to hold his hand as it rested on her shoulder.

The couple stayed like that for a considerable amount of time. Without needing me to cue him, he kept repeating softly to her, "I am here for you. I will do whatever it takes to keep you safe. I will never leave you." Her face and body melted. It was as if she was releasing a tension that had become built into her personality.

When she finally opened her eyes, she was a different person. She softly thanked her husband for doing this for her. Once they returned to the couch, the conversational dynamics shifted. He did most of the talking—explaining how important his wife was to him and how he did not want her to suffer. She was quiet and just kept looking into his eyes.

I sought commitment by asking her, "Do you believe now that he truly loves you?" With a look of slight embarrassment, she said that she knew he loved her.

It was as if a spell had been broken. Following that session, no further couples counseling was sought.

When seeking to use imaginative involvement for a reimagined past, keep in mind that your actual task is to help create a better future. Or, if it is the future that is to be reimagined, then make it clear to the client that this is a virtual reality in which anything is possible. As with a child who is invited to paint a self-portrait, "reality" is less material than creativity. Self-organized change and the emotional experience of choice is enhanced when the client is placed in the lead of the creative process. If the imagery summoned in therapy is emotionally powerful, then it will help redefine unconscious thought and emotion. As a rule, endeavor to keep autobiographical memories consistent, leaving the basic gist of the story intact. Powerful therapy can be achieved just by changing the interpretative details (reframing) or the emotional experience (counter-regulation). As one's internal reality expands through creative endeavors, so will the opportunities to externally express one's new reality.

10.3 Goal-pursuit

Any meaningful goal is infused with emotion and thereby a motivating force that summons a prescribed set of thoughts, habits, and instinctual actions. The interdependent actions of choice and automaticity move in and out of the spotlight of conscious deliberation. Internally, we experiment with these future actions as we imagine achieving the goal or failing to do so. As William James reasoned, this use of imagined outcomes enables us to test our ideas in virtual space. In James's (1912, 61) words, "By experimenting on our ideas of reality, we may save ourselves the trouble of experimenting on the real experiences which they severally mean." This is perhaps one of the most important capabilities of human intelligence.

Whenever a therapist helps a person imagine his or her preferred future and the obstacles that need to be overcome, it is referred to as mental contrasting. If the client is presenting with an anxious or depressed state, then he or she is most likely imagining a future filled with negative outcomes. The therapeutic task is to engage the positive half of this virtual reality. If the client begins to establish plans for how to achieve the desired outcome, this serves as a motivational catalyst and intellectual focal point.

For unconscious process work, the aim is to invoke an emotional image so compelling that the use of the words "planning" or "goal" is unnecessary. Even better is to recognize and access a system of values so central to the client's identity that they transcend the finite nature of his or her existence.

You can experience what I mean by imagining yourself sitting in your office with an elderly couple sitting across from you. The wife looks worried, and the husband is clearly unhappy to be in your office. With his arms crossed and his gaze set on you in a defiant manner, he explains, "It was not my idea to go see a therapist. I'm only here because my wife thinks it will help, and the doctors at Mayo gave us your name."

When the husband finishes his announcement, his wife apologetically explains her intentions,

> I am worried about my husband. He is seriously depressed. He hardly eats any food and spends most of his time in a dark bedroom. I have never seen him like this. He has always been such a good father and caring husband, but now he has stopped talking to our adult children and is not spending any time with his grandchildren.

At this point, he interrupts, "Do you want to tell him why I am depressed or should I?"

As the therapy expert, you speak up, "I think it would be best if you [the man] tell your own story." This is his response,

> I have spent all my life solving problems and being a leader for our family. If ever my wife or any of our children were in trouble, they would come to me, and I would find a solution. I have never depended on anyone else for help, frankly, because it has never been needed. I have been healthy and strong up until now. But after having problems with fatigue and pain, I go to Mayo Clinic, where they supposedly have the best doctors in the world. They tell me that I have advanced pancreatic cancer. They inform me that I have, at best, a few months left to live. Then they tell me to come talk to you so that I am not depressed. Now you tell me this, what are you going to do for me that none of these other doctors can do? Are you able to cure cancer?

What is your response? Do you defend your profession and try to explain what benefits he can reasonably expect from therapy? Do you focus on the marriage, the family, or focus on his individual needs? More importantly, how would you initiate unconscious process work? Before reading further, give yourself a little time to see what stands out about this person.

My understanding of the situation was that this man had laid down a challenge. If I did not prove my worth within the first few moments of the meeting, I imagined he would tune me out for the rest of the session and never return.

This was a person who was used to being in charge. However, if I left him in charge of the therapeutic process, he would lead all three of us into his depression. Thus, my task was to rapidly out-dominate this man, but I could not do so by trying to offer advice. Nor would it help to try and encourage him to be more optimistic.

For him, I was a naïve stranger, no older than one of his sons, and since I was not facing death, I would have no right to offer any advice. As Erickson warns, "You're not telling the subject to 'do this or do that.' So many therapists tell their patients how to think and how to feel. That is awfully wrong" (Erickson et al., 1976, 101).

My experience with clients, and people in general, is that when you are uncertain of what behaviors they will find acceptable, it is best to respond with social mimicry. Because he had just challenged me, I replied with my own stern challenge (also ending in a question, as he had),

> Looking at you, I can see you are a leader and a strong person. You did not need to tell me that. My guess is that your children have never had to doubt whether their father is there to help them face their challenges and how to make the most of the life they have been given. I imagine that in the eyes of your grandchildren you are almost mythical—the person that their mommy and daddy look to for advice. [Before continuing, I wait for him to unconsciously nod in agreement.] So now I have a question for you. Would you rather focus your thoughts and energies on yourself and your impending death, or would you like to turn your attention back to your family and to their needs? What do you think will be most meaningful to you—to focus on yourself or on the greatest challenge your family has ever had to face?

He replied that he had always been a servant leader—someone who dedicated his life to taking care of others rather than focusing on his own selfish interest. Now his voice had softened and no longer seemed condescending. He sounded sincere when he asked, "What can I do for my family … now that I have this disease?" With his eyes starting to tear, he confessed, "I've never felt so powerless." This is when I helped him shift to goal-oriented thinking, without using the term,

> You have no choice but to face death, eventually. Of the three of us sitting in this room, you are most likely to encounter death first. But someday, I will die as well. And, so will your beloved wife. Although we all hope it will be a long time from now, each of your three children will also

> have to face death. It is something that can be done poorly, in a state of despair and panic, or it can be done nobly and with gratitude for all the goodness you have experienced during your time on earth. You see, *you are leading your family into death.* The lessons you teach will potentially carry forward for generations. If you do this right, your great grandchildren and great-great grandchildren will benefit from the strength and leadership of a man they discover in stories from their parents. My question to you is: Are you going to let depression stand in the way of this achievement? If not, then what do you need to do differently when you return to home?

He had been gazing at me in a state of intense interest. After a moment of silence, he said,

> When I came here, I did not think you were going to be able to tell me anything that I did not already know. But you have said some things that I have not thought about before. [long pause] I am going to need to think about this for a while.

I agreed with his statement and pointed out that his mind would probably be working on a meaningful response even if he focused on other things, such as enjoying his wife and playing with his grandchildren.

His wife had a few questions for me about what she should do to support him. I essentially told her to be the same loving wife she has always been. He approved of this response, and then reasserted his dominance,

> I will come back to your office because you clearly have some valuable things to say. But I want some time in-between visits to work this out for myself. I think I will be ready to see you again in three weeks.

I replied that this sounded like the right amount of time to let his thoughts incubate.

Three weeks later when he and his wife returned his mood was greatly improved. The couple entered my office holding hands. Right away, the wife announced that she was happy to have her old husband back. She said that he had returned to interacting with family members in a loving, fun way.

He smiled an embarrassed smile and said that he had been caught off guard and needed a little assistance getting over the depression. After spending some time on pleasant small talk, he thanked me for helping him see the big picture and then said that he felt like he could handle his death moving forward and therefore did not need any further therapy. I told him he was the one who would know best what he needs, and *if* the symptoms of depression returned, *then* I would be here for him. He thanked me and apparently did not need any further psychological help.

When seeking to use mental contrasting in your own practice, keep in mind that you are not attempting to solve the client's problems, nor are you trying to arrive at a fixed state (a cure). Rather, you help engage natural problem-solving processes that move the client in a new, more productive direction. This is achieved in part by helping clients discover what goals matter most to them and what plans they can implement. This activity summons images of the future, with positive outcomes contrasted against negative outcomes, as well as images of past failures and lessons learned. While some of this mental activity may be explicit, and therefore verbalized to the therapist, the majority will necessarily take place outside of conscious awareness (capacity principle).

As you begin to envision yourself helping others in your future, it is useful to recall the words of Carl Rogers (1961):

> It seems to me that the good life is not any fixed state. It is not, in my estimation, a state of virtue, or contentment, or nirvana, or happiness. It is not a condition in which the individual is adjusted, fulfilled, or actualized. … The good life is a process, not a state of being.
>
> (186)

As all of nature evolves, so does each individual life. This ongoing process of problem solving leads us to new, higher ideals. Thus, as a rule, healthy consciousness is always moving forward towards *new opportunities*—never stuck in a fleeting moment of achievement.

10.4 Insight

As a final exercise, imagine this: What if someone handed you a piece of paper, which you would carry with you for the next ten years, and on that paper was a message so profound that it had the potential to help you put into motion your most important life accomplishments. Now imagine that you are the therapist seeking to provide one of your clients with just such a thing. You have only got one shot at this, so how do you ensure that the message you have given to your client is the right one? Relax into a few moments of creative speculation and see what comes to mind.

I mention this because I was asking myself that exact same question as I prepared to work with a volunteer in front of a large audience. I had been scheduled for a hypnosis demonstration at the 2011 International Congress on Ericksonian Approaches to Hypnosis and Psychotherapy. But I was personally interested in the question of insight and how this might be achieved unconsciously while using projectives.

A few hours before I was scheduled to go on stage, a young woman approached me and volunteered to be a demonstration subject. She said she was eager to work with me but nervous about what she might discover about herself in an auditorium filled with people. I assured her that her emotional work would be so private that not only would the audience not know, but much of it could also remain unknown to her own conscious awareness.

At the time, she was a graduate student uncertain of what career to pursue. Much later, I learned that while she was young her mother had become psychotic, and she had become terrified that she too was going crazy. She could not feel emotions, could not sustain relationships, and was wondering if she had a schizoaffective disorder.

During the demonstration, after helping her feel at ease and then deeply absorbed in her inner experiences, I invited her to close her eyes and see a piece of paper. I told her that the paper was blank and that she would write two very important messages on that paper, but she probably would not be able to see what she wrote. In order to help her become more deeply involved with this imagery, I instructed her to write using her non-dominant hand.

A year later, she came to see me at my office to continue her work. I was happy to be able to continue our collaboration. Her visits continued with approximately six months between each session over the course of nine years. Each year, I witnessed her becoming stronger and more self-assured. A few weeks ago, she met with me for her twentieth visit.

By this time, she had become an established therapist in private practice and a successful government consultant. Now feeling confident, emotionally alive, and about to be married, she spent much of the session describing how eager she was to start a family with her future husband. This was new. Becoming a mother was something she had previously imagined to be psychologically out of reach.

During this visit she said,

> You know, that piece of paper must still be traveling around with me in my unconscious. It keeps turning up in my dreams just before I take some major step forward in my life. Often, I am carrying it and showing it to others. But I still do not know what is on the note. But last night, I handed the piece of paper to my mother and my brother. They received it in the way they were supposed to. [pause] I had the feeling of the letter accomplishing what it was meant to accomplish.

I mention this case to inspire our appreciation for how deeply impacted someone can be by insights that are not fully known to conscious awareness. As the saying goes: "Give a man a fish, and he is fed for a day. But teach the man to fish, and he is fed for a lifetime." Similarly, the best type of insight to achieve in therapy is the type that helps sustain a lifetime of more effective problem solving. As a rule, do not attempt to remedy a client's problems with your solutions. Instead, create opportunities for people to learn more about their unconscious competencies and how to trust their own inspired solutions.

10.5 Healthy Consciousness

Like our body, if we think of the mind as having different parts that serve different functions, then unconscious intelligence is the metaphorical hands and feet. This is the part of mind most capable of producing adaptive behavior as it responds rapidly to the environment. There are countless examples of people acting to protect their lives or save someone else's without any thought.

In contrast, conscious intelligence functions as the eyes of this metaphorical body, enabling the mind to carefully monitor the effects of behavior on the environment. As evidence of this function, think of science as a highly developed use of conscious attention (such as when using symbolic logic or abstract math to study outcomes) and how good this use of conscious intelligence is at predicting the effect of our actions on the environment.

After seeing all the research that shows how ill-equipped conscious awareness is for introspection, it becomes clear that, like a pair of eyes, ordinary conscious attention is most wisely invested in a study of the external world.[2] Conscious awareness functions best when used to monitor concrete events, as with strategic planning or detailed evaluations.

When I help construct strategic plans for clients to think about (consciously), they express gratitude for "the tools" I am giving them. In everyday life we use tools to achieve practical ends somewhere outside of ourselves. This is the secret to utilization—to focus conscious attention *externally*, on some task that has emotional meaning or practical value, while incorporating automatic behavior(s) and implicit learning (Short 2020).

The reason for managing conscious attention this way is clearly illustrated in sports. For example, a study by Robin Jackson and colleagues (2006) found that athletes perform better when their attention is focused on external action rather than internal processes. In other words, rather than focusing conscious awareness on the mechanics of their bodies, successful athletes focus on strategic end goals, such as where to hit the ball or which person to block. Focusing on the environment and the effects one wishes to have on it (explicit goals) seems to be the best use of conscious awareness.

In contrast, *internal ends seem to be best suited to unconscious process work.* When we seek to use the conscious part of the mind to regulate deep internal states, which it does not have full access to, we not only set ourselves up for problems, such as confabulation and ironic rebound, but we also sacrifice mental energy that could have been utilized by adaptive unconscious processes. This does not mean that unconscious intelligence is superior; rather, each form of processing serves different purposes.

According to Dijksterhuis and Nordgren's (2016) *capacity principle*, the choice of either conscious or unconscious resources should be determined by the type of mental processing that is needed. Skillful problem solvers do not expect their conscious faculties to perceive and process more than the limits of ability. Nor do they rely exclusively on intuition. For optimal use of mental ability, we need a discerning engagement of conscious and unconscious intelligence.

In contrast to conscious awareness, unconscious processes are better suited for monitoring the effects of the environment on our internal states of being. Thus, people are encouraged to "trust their gut" on complex decisions, and having done so, the outcomes are typically superior to those of conscious calculation. The person may say, "I don't know why, but for some reason this does not feel right to me." The reason is because unconscious processes have subliminally picked up on information or tapped into memories that conscious awareness does not have access to.

We should appreciate the fact that an unconscious search accesses far more information than is consciously available. As a rule, when faced with highly complex problems, such as deciding who to marry, we should create as much time as possible for deep processing. We can do this by asking ourselves the question that needs to be answered and then waiting for the answer to be formulated outside of conscious awareness. As we continue to ask ourselves the same question, we should pay special attention to our dreams or look for "signs" during everyday activities that have an unusual emotional impact. We can also use prayer, meditation, or self-hypnosis to remain focused on the problem while still maintaining a state of conscious surrender.

As an additional rule, when the stakes are high and rapid responding is important, we should allow ourselves to act rather than cogitate. Our unconscious intelligence has instant access to survival instincts and practiced skill sets that manifest in purposeful, coordinated action, even before there is time to think. When other therapists ask me, "How do you think so fast during therapy?" I often reply, "I don't think. I act. And, if I do not have any urge to act upon, then I sit back and collect more information." This boundless problem-solving cycle—act … assess … act … assess—means that I am never at a loss for what to do.

During therapy, the therapist's unconscious attention is most wisely invested in a study of the internal workings of the client's mental landscape. This will produce "spontaneous" behavior that is uniquely inspirational or motivational. It is a provocative form of therapy that does not seek to provide concrete answers but instead asks the right questions. The provocation might come in the form of a poignant story, subtle humor, a symbolic act, an evocative gesture, the use of metaphor or analogies—anything that acts as a catalyst for emotional fluidity (seeing things from a different emotional perspective) and automaticity (any process that is not under the control of conscious intention).

The procedures described in this book are useful guides that will enable you to achieve beneficial outcomes with those who come to you for help. Ideally, you should experiment with these techniques at the first available opportunity to help solidify your learning and build confidence. As you learn how to use the technique, remain equally aware of why it has value.

A good technique is like a roadway that provides a reasonably straight path to a desired destination. However, the principles that orient us to the value of each technique form the foundations of good clinical judgement. Thus, just as compass directions tell us which roads to travel and why, the principles in this book help navigate the twists and turns of strategically tailored psychotherapy.

At the beginning of this book, you were primed to learn underlying principles rather than focusing primarily on techniques. As the therapist expert, it is your responsibility to know the end to which therapy should progress. The principles described in this book are meant to collectively chart a course towards greater mental health.

In summary, the overarching principle that frames the practical value of each of these techniques is growth-oriented problem solving, which is synonymous with establishing a growth mindset. Just as all of nature continues to evolve, so must each individual life.

Using this broad concept, we can delineate some essential activities of healthy consciousness, such as motivation, creativity (with humor and imaginative play), choice, and goal-oriented striving that is guided by one's own profound insights. These activities respectively produce the subjective experiences of hopeful purpose, generative thriving, freedom, joyful intelligence, and self-efficacy. Other essential experiences, such as the giving and receiving of love, cooperative collaboration, and gentle humor, are byproducts of healthy relationships that hopefully characterize the way you conduct your life as well as the practice of therapy. It is also the spirit in which I have endeavored to share with you my highest ideals.

Notes

1 Psychotherapy has an unfortunate history of labeling angry women as victims of rape. Those with no such memory have been subjected to theories of memory repression at the risk of implanting false memories. This is unethical. A recent report from the CDC (2020) states that one in five women will experience attempted or completed sexual assault during their lifetime. So, we should not be surprised if as many as 20% of female clientele report sexual trauma. But for the other 80% percent, we need to recognize the countless other ways the psyche can be damaged.

2 Accordingly, sciences like psychology and neurology are NOT introspective. They focus the scientists' conscious attention on external realities, such as brain scans and behavioral outcomes. Ironically, we learn most about the internal workings of the mind by studying it from the outside.

References

CDC. 2020. "Sexual Assault Awareness." *Centers for Disease Control and Prevention.* May 1. http://www.cdc.gov/injury/features/sexualviolence.

Dijksterhuis, Ap, and Loran F. Nordgren. 2016. "A Theory of Unconscious Thought:" *Perspectives on Psychological Science* 1 (2): 95–109. doi:10.1111/j.1745-6916.2006.00007.x.

Erickson, Milton H., Ernest L. Rossi, and Sheila I. Rossi. 1976. "Hypnotic Realities: The Induction of Clinical Hypnosis and Forms of Indirect Suggestion." In *Hypnotic Realities: The Induction of Clinical Hypnosis and Forms of Indirect Suggestion.* Vol. 10. Phoenix, AZ: Milton H. Erickson Foundation Press.

Jackson, Robin C., Kelly J. Ashford, and Glen Norsworthy. 2006. "Attentional Focus, Dispositional Reinvestment, and Skilled Motor Performance under

Pressure." *Journal of Sport and Exercise Psychology* 28 (1): 49–68. doi:10.1123/jsep.28.1.49.

James, William. 1912. *Essays in Radical Empiricism*. Edited by Ralph Barton Perry. New York: Longmans, Green, & Co. Project Gutenberg. http://www.gutenberg.org/ebooks/32547.

Rogers, Carl Ransom. 1961. *On Becoming a Person: A Therapist's View of Psychotherapy*. New York: Houghton Mifflin.

Short, Dan. 2020. *From William James To Milton Erickson: The Care of Human Consciousness*. New York: Archway Publishing.

Index

For Product Safety Concerns and Information please contact our EU
representative GPSR@taylorandfrancis.com
Taylor & Francis Verlag GmbH, Kaufingerstraße 24, 80331 München, Germany

www.ingramcontent.com/pod-product-compliance
Ingram Content Group UK Ltd.
Pitfield, Milton Keynes, MK11 3LW, UK
UKHW022313250926
475702UK00046B/756
9780367649678